Robert Fulford, D.O. and the
Philosopher Physician

# Robert Fulford, D.O.
## *and the*
# Philosopher Physician

Zachary Comeaux, D.O., F.A.A.O.

EASTLAND PRESS · SEATTLE

Published by Eastland Press, Incorporated
P.O. Box 99749, Seattle, WA 98199  USA

International Standard Book Number:  0-939616-36-X
Library of Congress Control Number:  2002102917

The design for the background of the cover and first page of each chapter is based on Walter Russell's depiction of the "cosmic pendulum."

2  4  6  8  10  9  7  5  3  1

Book and cover design by Gary Niemeier

# Table of Contents

# TABLE OF CONTENTS

# Foreword

*"You're not responding as well as I had hoped;*
*I'm going to have to use something stronger.*
*This is twenty-first century medicine."*

I heard the late Robert C. Fulford, D.O., F.C.A., utter these words as I lay on the treatment table in his home at Waverly, Ohio in April of 1994. I had sought his help because I had not been recovering well from an acute illness which had begun several months earlier. "Doc," as I affectionately called him, showed me a case containing three crystals of varying strength. In the course of treatment, he used two of these crystals before I began to respond satisfactorily, so that he could resume his customary treatment pattern. I then began to respond more and more to his use of palpatory assessment, interpretation, and the oscillatory effects of the percussion vibrator. The third crystal was never used in my treatment, and by October of 1996, thanks to his ministrations, I finally recovered my sense of improved health and respiratory effectiveness. Doctor Fulford passed on the following year.

During the course of his professional life, Doc contributed to osteo-pathic thought and served as a guide to the development of that thought among the osteopathic physicians who will follow him. The patients in whom health was restored through his love, practice, and thought will always be grateful.

Zachary J. Comeaux, D.O., F.A.A.O., the author of this text, is partic-ularly well situated to understand the significance of Dr. Fulford's work. He was a frequent companion of Doc's during the final years of his life. As a physician to the late Mrs. Fulford, and with access to Dr. Fulford's notebooks, papers, and source books in the months following his death, Dr. Comeaux offers an expanded view of his thought and methods. I have known and worked with Dr. Comeaux since the years of his predoctoral program at the Ohio University College of Osteopathic Medicine (OUCOM). It has been my privilege to know him as a student, friend, and colleague on the school faculty.

The physiologic premises underlying Dr. Fulford's work and thought are examined by the author in both historical and contemporary contexts. This approach reveals that aspects of neuroproprioceptive physiology and tonic vibratory reflex are not generally applied in the clinic. It facilitates an understanding of Dr. Fulford's elaboration of the thought of Andrew Taylor Still, M.D., D.O., and William Garner Sutherland, D.O., as well as those aspects which are unique to Dr. Fulford.

Doc made his last professional appearance at the 1997 Cranial Academy Convention in Chicago. There he pleaded with his audience to rely on osteopathy to better understand the complex streams of moving energy of which our patients are comprised. The author's effort in writ-ing this book addresses that plea.

Anthony G. Chila, D.O., F.A.A.O.
Professor, Department of Family Medicine
Ohio University College of Osteopathic Medicine
Athens, Ohio

# Introduction

Throughout his life as a healer, Robert Fulford, D.O., was variously perceived as being an innovative, controversial, and charismatic figure. At a time when factions debated the case for alternative versus conventional evidence-based medicine, and some suggested that osteopathic treatment and philosophy had become irrelevant, Robert Fulford inspired many students and practitioners to take another look at our basic assumptions about life, human nature, and health care. And in an era when the osteopathic community was mired in divisions over personal and regional preferences for certain techniques and terminology, Fulford explored and then integrated exciting ideas into his osteopathic treatment approach. He always believed that this was in the true spirit of Drs. Still and Sutherland, his osteopathic elders.

Working within the tradition of cranial osteopathy, Fulford presented his ideas at convocations of the American Academy of Osteopathy, and at conventions of The Cranial Academy. In 1998, the year after his death, the AAO dedicated its convocation to Fulford's work. A book containing his papers and speeches will be published by The Cranial Academy.

Robert Fulford was a practical dreamer. He relied on intuition, but studied furiously, gleaning ideas from ancient religions, philosophy, poetry, astrology, physics, and other sources to develop practical guidelines for the clinic and for life. He contended that medicine unnecessarily limited its success by focusing its attention on the physical aspect of the patient. He urged that more attention be paid to the etheric or energetic body— what he called "energy medicine" and "twenty-first century medicine." While this idea is integral to many ancient traditions, western physiology and physics have only just begun to make the connection.

Robert Fulford taught that "thoughts are things" which can hurt or heal; that love and service are essential elements of care and treatment; that the key to current symptoms lies in the previous life experiences of the patient; and that the hands can be used to treat on a physical, emotional, and spiritual level. But beyond all this, he gave hope and health to many individuals previously considered untreatable. As his reputation grew, he treated both his neighbors and those from around the globe. Disabled from birth, or carrying deep emotional scars which surfaced as pain, many were led to more comfortable, functional lives through his gentle but forceful words and touch. At bottom, he thought of himself as a catalyst for change in the ongoing development of the patient.

No book can capture the expressions, private thoughts, gestures, or the auric presence of an individual. Moreover, Fulford's life was an intellectual journey in which ideas flowed like a swift current, and no one set of concepts embodied his thought. Fulford never undertook the task of writing a textbook for the profession. He felt that the finality of the printed word failed to represent the complexity and multifaceted nature of his evolving thought—his work was never complete enough to suit him. Because of the limited resources available to a practicing physician, he did very little formal research or publishing. Yet he was universally admired as an insightful and incisively effective clinician.

In writing the popular book *Dr. Fulford's Touch of Life*, intended as a sampler, not a textbook, Fulford asked me and others for assistance with the project. Later, in the months following his death, I stored his books and papers at my home before they were distributed according to his will.

It was an exciting experience for me to sort through his papers, retracing the path of his intellectual life and discovering the sources of the ideas that he tried to unify and express.

I had the opportunity to join Dr. Fulford on a number of personal and professional journeys, and to care for his wife in a nursing home near my office during the last years of her life. Fulford often visited my office. Each visit would begin with my question, "Well, what are you thinking about this week?" Sometimes we would work on each other. Sometimes we would see patients together. His mind was always investigating and reflecting.

Since his passing I have assimilated most of what he left on paper, plowing through stacks of saved material, including notebooks and course materials, and reading the works of the writers who influenced him, many of whom are not described elsewhere. In preparing this book, I have tried to strike a balance between presenting the material as it was taught by Dr. Fulford, and elaborating upon it, based on his source materials themselves.

This book includes practical applications of techniques, and attention to an expanded sense of palpatory awareness and its use in treatment. Fulford's way of expressing all of this was not as abstract as mine. He was a very practical man; his thoughts were organized in a dissociated, eclectic, Zen-like manner. By contrast, I have tried to express the expansive worldview that he brought to the osteopathic treatment table in a more linear fashion. Some redundancy in the text will hopefully serve to reinforce the concentric nature of Fulford's thought in practice, emphasizing different nuances at different times, just as the same notes in music serve as the basis for a variety of melodies.

Dr. Fulford fought for what he believed, but in a gentle way. What is more, he also fought with himself over issues of intellectual pride and self-promotion. However, it was always with a reverence for the pursuit of truth, including scientific explanation, and for the broader role of participating in the divine creative process. He saw medicine as a practice of loving service, not one of control, wealth, or pride of accomplishment. He always saw himself as part of an evolving osteopathic community of understanding.

INTRODUCTION

It is hoped that this book will fill a gap in the resources available to those of us who are trying to preserve, teach, and pass on the insights and methods of this wonderful man. None of us can ever truly speak for Dr. Fulford, or treat just as he would have with his own hands, heart, and mind. We can only learn from him to enrich our own paths.

• • •

I would like to thank The Cranial Academy for the opportunity to utilize Dr. Fulford's speeches and papers, which were bequethed to The Cranial Academy upon his death. His speeches and papers will be published by The Cranial Academy under the title *Are We on the Path? Collected Works of Robert C. Fulford, D.O., F.C.A.*

I am grateful to Dr. Fulford for befriending me and taking me as a student. I am also grateful to his wife, Glenna, for her patience with both of us. I would like to thank their sons, Richard and David, for their cooperation in this endeavor. Thanks also to my wife, Linda, for her patience. Finally, I am grateful to Anthony Chila, D.O., who as teacher and friend, as well as fellow student and patient of Dr. Fulford's, was instrumental in assisting me with the publication of this book.

There is a community of osteopathic students and physicians who have been touched by Dr. Fulford, and from whom this work springs. I am grateful to all of you for allowing me to be included in your company.

# PART ONE

## Introductory Material

"My object is to make the osteopath a philosopher, and place him on the rock of reason. Then I will not have to worry of writing details of how to treat any organ of the body, because he is qualified to the degree of knowing what has produced the variations of all kinds in form and function."

*—Andrew Taylor Still*

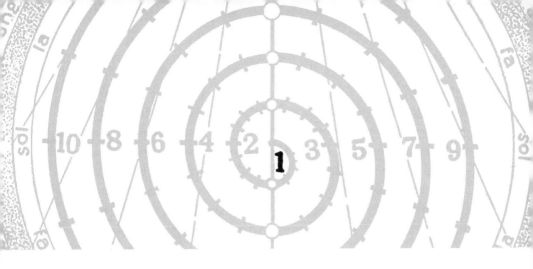

**1**

# Impact on the Profession

## The Challenge

*T*he selection of the work and thought of Robert Fulford, D.O., as the theme for the 1998 convocation of the American Academy of Osteopathy reflects the importance of this man to the osteopathic profession. As a frequent speaker before the AAO and The Cranial Academy, Dr. Fulford brought a new perspective to the definition of osteopathy and the osteopathic concept. To a profession that is questioning the relevance of its manual tradition, and is drifting toward a proliferation of models for its techniques, he refocused our attention on the importance of understanding the basic but multifaceted nature of the person in promoting health.

I stress the word *refocus* because Fulford's work makes much more sense in the context of questions raised by his osteopathic forebears. Those who do not look for this connection may see Fulford as a proponent of alternative or esoteric medicine. Admittedly, because of the inclusiveness of his thinking, he often categorized himself as such. However, as reflected in his personal history, Fulford's thought is grounded firmly in the evolving osteopathic philosophy of Andrew Taylor Still and William Garner Sutherland. The ideas of these pioneers of osteopathy are sometimes presented as finished works, but that is not the case. If we trace the development of their thought through their writings, we find that their ideas do not represent closed or defined systems. The challenge is therefore not simply to assimilate and implement these systems of thought. Rather, the development of their thought should be seen as a progressive quest into the deeper philosophical and spiritual questions underlying the nature of the person, which has practical implications for the form and manner of our techniques, as well as our demeanor and attitudes as practitioners. This quest is an essential part of being a technically effective clinician.

Fulford's work is based on a novel way of looking at the patient and the physician. In this chapter, we will trace:

- The relationship in osteopathic tradition between ideas and technique, supporting the primary importance of recognizing one's own philosophy
- The relationship of Fulford's philosophy to that of Still and Sutherland.

The premise is that a discussion of these topics, here and throughout the book, will lead to a progressive refinement of certain aspects of one's awareness, culminating in the adaptation of treatment methods suggested by Fulford.

William Sutherland described this process as "digging on," using the analogy of digging potatoes in a field. If you've ever done this, you know that once you've pulled the vines and dug the patch with a fork, you feel the satisfaction of a hard job done well. However, if you dig deeper or even go through the same depth again, you will find more potatoes. No matter how thoroughly you dig, nature will still reveal some volunteer sprouts from spuds that were hidden in the soil. So it is with understanding the implications of osteopathic findings in a patient.

## Fulford in the History of Osteopathic Philosophical Thought

Robert Fulford graduated in 1941 from the Kansas City School of Osteopathy and Surgery, where he had studied under the students of

Andrew Taylor Still. Soon after, he came under the influence of William Sutherland. From pressure to compete with allopathic physicians in general practice, he watched the drift of American osteopathy toward the medical model. However, just like Still and Sutherland before him, a spark enkindled an intellectual fire within him that would consume his life. He was, as Still encouraged his students to be, a philosopher physician.[1]

Fulford "dug on." He listened to the jargon about osteopathy treating the whole person, the interrelationship of structure and function, and the integration of body, mind, and spirit. Then he spent a life putting flesh onto these truisms by looking deeper into their meaning. His thought and methodology challenge us to rethink our approach to our work and the scope of osteopathy. He spoke of the ethric body, energy sinks, taking out the shock, and a "flip" in the tissue.[2] He recommended that we look upon thoughts as things, and that we treat by intention, concepts that are elaborated later in this text.[3] These ideas seem foreign to present-day osteopathic thinking; however, they make more sense in the context of the unanswered questions of his (and our) osteopathic predecessors. The question of where to put "appropriate," correct, or effective techniques has been around since the early days of osteopathy.

It should be recalled that it was twenty years after Dr. Still named his art before he attempted to teach others. And even then, if you read his work, you will see that he struggled for the rest of his life to define the essence of osteopathy. He intentionally declined to write a treatment manual. His closest effort, *Osteopathy Research and Practice*, included the following comment:

> My object is to make the osteopath a philosopher, and place him on the rock of reason. Then I will not have to worry of writing details of how to treat any organ of the body, because he is qualified to the degree of knowing what has produced the variations of all kinds in form and function.[4]

The essence of Still's writing is concerned with the restoration of anatomic order based on the premise that the order of the body represents the law of nature, which in turn reflects the work of the all-knowing Creator. The extent to which an individual is functional or dysfunctional is a reflection of their relative harmony with the nature of man, as created by God. In a curious lecture/sermon delivered in 1895, Still likened his own quest for knowledge to a search for the divine mystery of nature:

> The first discovery I made was this: that every single individual stroke of God came to me as unknowable. The stroke of death—what do you know about this? I know nothing, therefore it is unknowable. I began to study and experiment.[5]

Still went on to imply that he always tried to read the intended order in the body, partly by being familiar with its anatomy. We usually understand this to mean the identification and cataloging of the body's parts, and their structural and functional relationships. While this is surely part of what he intended, Still implied that he was more directed by intuitively yielding to the sense of harmony imposed by the Creator as a reflection of the individual's state of health.

Andrew Still loved and ardently preached the study of anatomy as an empiric science, as reflected in the following passage: "Therefore, let me work with that body, from the brain to the feet. It is all finished work, and is trustworthy in all its parts."[6] Nevertheless, he implied many times in his works that correct thinking came from intuition, illuminated by reason. Sometimes the practitioner, in a moment of insight, would make a leap in seeing and understanding patterns in the body. Still's experiential analogy of the Ram of Reason—the sudden intrusion of a critical insight while dreaming—conveyed the force, cogency, and spontaneity of such new ideas.[7]

## Expanded Scope of Osteopathic Work

As a student, Fulford heard about this idea of looking for the expanded sense of order that included the articular anatomy and palpable physiology. In 1945 he allowed himself to be drawn to Still's work as elaborated by William Sutherland. Dr. Sutherland was struggling to express the unification of body, mind, and spirit in his own work. His inspired insight into the significance of the sphenoid articulations of the cranium led to an understanding of the interrelationship of structure and function that was expressed in the subtle relationships among the membranes, bones, and fluids in the rest of the body. But more than that, Sutherland's appreciation of the individual patient as part of a creative act—the gift of life itself—infiltrated all of his thinking.

Sutherland's work emphasized an idea of Still's: "Life is matter in motion."[8] Sutherland spent a lifetime reflecting upon and explaining the significance of this motion that he initially experienced in the cranium, where gross, voluntary motion was at a minimum. Throughout his life he continued to elucidate, as it became clearer to him, that there was a relationship between the anatomy and quality of motion in a patient and his state of health, which in turn reflected the extent to which the individual was in harmony with the intent of the Creator. He made it clear that this knowledge, which he appreciated and passed on, did not come from learning or research, but was divinely inspired.[9] Sutherland's integration of spirituality with clinical practice is well summarized in the work of another of his students, Rollin Becker.[10] This theme represents a significantly less tangible dimension than the anatomic one.

Still and Sutherland were not unique in trying to reconcile the empiric and esoteric spheres of reality. This apparent dichotomy has plagued every generation that has struggled to improve the quality of human life. In our own day, materialism appears to have an upper hand over vitalism in the arena of health science. Yet those of us who believe in Still's admonition to integrate the Triune aspects of man in our approach to medicine continue to struggle with how to do it.

Fulford joined the cranial osteopathic movement during a time when it was struggling for recognition and scientific legitimacy. That was a time, during Sutherland's latter days, when the preoccupation was with the validation and recognition of the measurability of cranial movement, the articular relationships that made this possible, and the amplitude of pressure changes that would explain the fluid wave or "tide" as transmitted by the cerebrospinal fluid. The physiological importance of these things to the health and well-being of the individual was stressed. It was a formidable challenge that was nobly (and successfully) undertaken by many of Sutherland's disciples: Ann Wales, Rollin Becker, Beryl Arbuckle, Harold Magoun, Rebecca and Harold Lippincott, and Viola Frymann. The success of the cranial approach can be gauged by the extent to which this concept has been adapted and integrated into bodywork worldwide. It represents another dimension of the human organism, and another effective method for restoring health.

Yet when—following his admonition to dig on—we read the later writings of Sutherland, we can see that he was struggling with deeper insights that challenged description. We are familiar with his invocation of Still's comment about the cerebrospinal fluid being the highest known element.[11] Yet in talks, he spoke of "Liquid Light" as a higher level in the cascade of causes defining life. He described the "potency" within the cerebrospinal fluid as a fluid within a fluid, and he used the image of a glass house illuminated by the refraction of light flowing through it to show its form. Just so in the patient, where the quality of movement of the cerebrospinal fluid reflects the state of the person's health. Sutherland suggested that a palpable vital force was discernible in the body's subtle movements, including that of the cerebrospinal fluid.[12]

We see in these ideas a need to go beyond conventional—including cranioarticular—anatomy and physiology. Where was he going? In this text, we will explore Fulford's role in the philosophical questions that form the backbone of osteopathic thought.

Dr. Fulford appreciated Sutherland's expansion of the scope of osteopathic practice beyond a biomechanical, articular model. In his Percussion Vibrator courses, when describing the nature of the person, Fulford referred to the analogy of the glass house.[13] He went back into what Still called "the unknowable" from a different point of view, enriched by his contact with Sutherland. He recognized that one must return to the fundamentals in order to understand the nature of a patient and thereby appreciate the significance of his or her complaint. In so doing, he was reaching with Still and Sutherland beyond the tangible aspect of the person toward an expanded insight.

## Redefining the Patient

### Energetic Dimensions

An early insight of Fulford's led him to emphasize the electromagnetic aspect of motion in defining life. As an undergraduate student in osteopathic school he had communicated with Harold Saxton Burr, a Yale neurophysiologist who did work on measuring the "life field," initially in trees, but later in comparative studies between healthy women and those with uterine cancer. Burr described the life field as a measurable, low amplitude direct current phenomenon. Fulford spent much of the rest of his life trying to correlate theoretical models, scientific measurement, diagnostic significance, and intervention strategies based on the existence of this life field as an aspect of the individual's constitution. He felt that this was an extension of the functional concepts of Sutherland and of Still's notions regarding the Triune nature of man and the biogenic life force. Fulford thereby described a new paradigm for osteopathic thought that resonates with many of us today.

Fulford's practice style evolved throughout his life. In its final form, his methods were unconventional and outside the mainstream of osteopathy. They included, for example,

- Articular and structural analysis, but with a subtle turning of attention concurrently to the ethric body
- Connective tissue analysis when he was interested in the respiratory response, but with refined attention to the developmental causes and consequences of the quality of the breath.

In difficult cases, direct manipulation of the ethric body through intention, percussive vibration, crystals, or magnetic devices was employed.

At the 1997 convention of The Cranial Academy, where Fulford presented the final and fullest expression of his thought, he made the point that unless osteopathy included the energetic approach, the elaboration of truth about the nature of the human person would become the province of others. He treated Margaret Sorrel, D.O., using a newly devised protocol based on the work of Norm Sheally and Carolyn Myss, but with a Vogel cut quartz crystal.[14]

He was asked, "Do you have to be an osteopath to do this—this does not look very osteopathic?" to which he responded, "If I weren't an osteopath, how would I know what to do?" This succinct response reflected the fact that his approach to the patient was deeply grounded in osteopathic philosophy, tempered by his own reading, reflection, and integration of compatible, but more wide-ranging, concepts. What he meant was that he was guided by the osteopathic principles of body unity and the interrelationship of structure and function, although his application of these principles was unique. Soon after that meeting, he allowed the Breath of Life to take him elsewhere—he expired.

Thus, Fulford insisted that his approach represented legitimate inquiries into osteopathy and that he was building on the ideas of Still and Sutherland. He pursued his concept of the nature of man and the intelligent application of osteopathic principles in the context of two aspects of Still's thought: the Triune nature of man and the biogenic life force, both briefly discussed here and later in the text.

### Triune Man

Very often quoted, but a challenge to implement beyond the level of slogan, is the following passage from Still:

> First there is the material body, second the spiritual being, third a being of mind which is far superior to all vital motions and material forms, whose duty is to manage this great engine of life. This great principle known as mind must depend for all evidence on the five senses; on this testimony, all mental conclusions are made, and all orders from this mental court are issued to move to any point and stop at any place. Thus to obtain good results, we must blend ourselves with, and travel in harmony with, nature's truths.[15]

### Biogenic Life Force

Another line of thought of the mature Dr. Still were his reflections on the nature and manner of the operation of life, or the life force. He called this the Biogen. This concept is often ignored by those interested in going

10

directly to the theatre of treatment, bypassing the classroom of philosophy. As Still put it:

> What is life?
>
> If life in man were formed to suit the size and duties of the being, if life has a living and separate personage, then we should be governed by such reasons as would give it the greatest chance to go on with its labors in the bodies of men and of beasts. We know by experience that a spark of fire will start the principles of powder in motion, which, were it not simultaneous by the positive principle of Father nature, which finds this germ lying quietly in the womb of space, would be silently inactive for all ages. Without being able to move or help itself, save for the motor principle of life given from the Father of all motion.
>
> Right here we should ask the question "Is action produced by electricity put in motion, or is it the active principle that comes from spiritual man?"
>
> We see the form of each world, and call the united action biogenic life. All material bodies have life terrestrial and all space has life, ethereal or spiritual life. The two when united, form man.[16]
>
> His [the osteopath's] duty as a philosopher admonishes him that life and matter can be unified and that that union cannot continue with any hindrance to free and absolute motion.[17]

It is much easier to talk technique. However, there are implications in these musings that are relevant to physiology and that contain a message for those who would devise a technical approach to medicine. Fulford spent a lifetime elaborating on the notion that when we apply technique, successively deeper levels of effectiveness are attained based on the unification of our intention with the Divine creative process. The evidence for the existence of this process can be found in the layered complexity of the human person, of which an outer layer is the physical body, the object of study of classical anatomy. Fulford did not show *the* way; rather, he shared his experiments with truth.

## Food for the Journey

In 1945 Sutherland and Fulford visited with the artist, philosopher, and theoretical physicist Walter Russell. Russell was a systematic philosopher.

(One might recall the influence of Herbert Spencer, a systematic vitalist philosopher, on Still.[18]) Russell's cosmology tended to favor the Platonic view in which the physical world is seen as the manifestation of a higher order of reality. He theorized that reality was characterized by ordered, periodic motion and that discussions among physicists regarding the nature of light (the wave-particle notion that formed the backbone of quantum mechanics) had broad applications to the nature of man and health. Light, he said, in addition to being a physical phenomenon, was the tangible expression of Divine thought. Light, in its aspect as wave, was also the highest manifestation of periodic motion. Thus, the periodic motion characteristics of the elements in the periodic table described not only their chemical nature, but also the nature of the gross bodies compounded from aggregates of these elements, thus reflecting their dual nature. In other words, motion was initiated by Creative thought and was constitutive of the material body.

*The person is a complex derived from material and energetic influences.* The human body can be analyzed not just on the basis of its chemical elements, as a catalogue of its organic compounds, but also according to the composite effect of the energetic aspects of the bonds and their inherent motion. In Russell's cosmology, light, with its material and energetic quantum characteristics, is a medium for physical creation, growth, or decline in function of the individual. Thoughts or intentions have material influences on the state of the person. The *intention* of the physician, including a loving disposition, is a force analogous to light, which can contribute to change in the physical constitution of the person. These ideas are rich in their implications, and, because of their influence on osteopathic thought, will be elaborated upon later in the text.

Sutherland and Russell (along with the young Fulford) conducted unpublished research in diagnosis and treatment in accordance with their views on the human person. Fulford saw these experiments as justification for his interest in the L-field, or Life Field, and as providing further meaning to the concept of the Breath of Life, as expressed by Sutherland. In addition, Fulford discerned another level of significance in the restriction of motion (known to osteopaths as somatic dysfunction) secondary to trauma.

These experiments led to a direction of thinking that expressed itself quietly in the work of Sutherland, for example, in his concepts of the Breath of Life, the Tide, and Liquid Light. They were also a challenge to those osteopaths whose primary concern was to prove the reality of cranial mobility in scientific terms, and for whom such questions as the effectiveness of intention, the emotional and spiritual evolution of the patient, and palpation of the energetic state were less pressing.

Fulford spent the rest of his life exploring the expression of these realities. His study was diverse and interdisciplinary, even intercultural. He was strongly influenced by the work of such scientists as Robert Becker and Valerie Hunt, and the psychologist John Diamond. Later we will discuss the particular ideas of these individuals that influenced Fulford to remodel his concept of osteopathy.

## Clinical Challenges: The Difficult Cases

Fulford and his primary teachers realized, as did Still, that successful osteopathic treatment, especially in difficult or unresponsive cases, could only be improved by delving deeper into the nature of the person. Minor and acute complaints could be treated in a simplified mechanical manner. But they recognized that current science could not adequately describe the nature of many problems of health and illness expressed by patients. They accepted that another approach to the deeper nature of man included the spiritual dimension, and that it was necessary to integrate wisdom from the philosophical arena as a complement to current scientific understanding. Expressions from other cultures about the nature of man were often useful. Many insights into human nature had been preserved in the ancient religious practices of these cultures. Fulford felt that this paralleled the preservation of knowledge in houses of religious learning in medieval Europe during periods of popular disinterest in truth. Our contemporary culture mirrors this sentiment in the areas of consciousness studies, subtle energy medicine, and complementary or alternative medicine, often enriched by an intercultural exchange of ancient wisdom, literature, and practice.

Following in this tradition, Robert Fulford spent a lifetime exploring, reflecting, and integrating these issues, in accordance with the admonishment of Dr. Still:

> We see in man, as we comprehend it, the attributes of Deity. We see the results of the action of mind, therefore a representation of the Mind of minds.[19]

> God is the Father of Osteopathy, and I am not ashamed of the child of His mind.[20]

## REFERENCES

1. Still AT. *The Philosophy and Mechanical Principles of Osteopathy.* Kirksville, MO: Osteopathic Enterprise, 1992 (orig. 1902): 20.

2. Fulford R. *Dr. Fulford's Touch of Life.* New York: Pocket Books, 1996: 22.

3. Ibid., 42.

4. Still AT. *Osteopathy Research and Practice.* Seattle: Eastland Press, 1992 (orig. 1910): 65.

5. Still AT. *Autobiography of A.T. Still.* Indianapolis, IN: American Academy of Osteopathy, 1981 (orig. 1897, 1908): 241.

6. Ibid., 248.

7. Ibid., 356.

8. Still, *Philosophy and Mechanical Principles of Osteopathy*, 257.

9. Sutherland WG. *Contributions of Thought.* Sutherland A, Wales A (eds.) Fort Worth, TX: Sutherland Cranial Teaching Foundation, 1967: 158.

10. Becker R. *Life in Motion: The Osteopathic Vision of Rollin Becker.* Rachel Brooks (ed.) Portland, OR: Rudra Press, 1997: 24.

11. Sutherland WG. *Teachings in the Science of Osteopathy.* Portland, OR: Rudra Press, 1990: 32.

12. Sutherland, *Contributions of Thought*, 243.

13. These courses, begun in 1988, were presented at many venues across the United States. Fulford's course notebooks were private, and the material was delivered orally, with selected handouts. I have copies of the notebooks (the originals are in the possession of The Cranial Academy) and cite them in this text as references.

14. Schealy N, Myss, C. The ring of fire and dhea: a theory for energetic restoration of adrenal reserves. *Subtle Energies and Energy Medicine*, 1996; 6(2):167.

15. Still AT. *Philosophy of Osteopathy*. Colorado Springs, CO: American Academy of Osteopathy, 1946 (orig. 1899): 26, 28.

16. Still, *The Philosophy and Mechanical Principles of Osteopathy*, 249–51.

17. Ibid., 250.

18. Trowbridge C. *Andrew Taylor Still 1828–1917*. Kirksville, MO: The Thomas Jefferson University Press, 1991.

19. Still, *Autobiography of A.T. Still*, 259.

20. Ibid., 254.

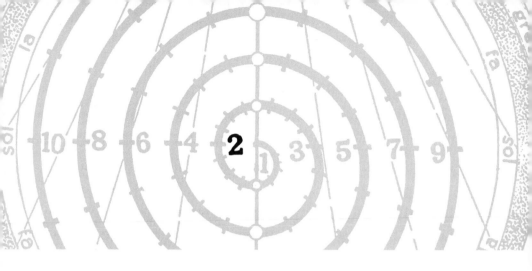

# The Materialist–Vitalist Dilemma: What is Life?

## Philosophy: A Background for Specific Knowledge

*W*e often use the term *philosophy* to describe the general concepts of Dr. Still and the early osteopaths. We noted in Chapter 1 that Still admonished his students to be philosophers and to become grounded in basic concepts around which we can organize our diagnoses and treatments.[1] However, the idea of a philosophy has a specific meaning, often lost to us in the present age.

In a remote time when men were basically humbled by what they did not understand about the world around them, they raised questions and postulated answers to unify their experiences. An ancient Greek would see an arrow fly and try to explain the reality behind the phenomenon. Did the perceptual change in the arrow during its trajectory represent a series of changes in the state of being of the arrow, some other attribute of the arrow, or a change in our point of view? There was an intuition that the *being* of an object, or person, was a special "something." A number of systematic ways of looking at the universe developed as an outgrowth of this inquiry. The field of inquiry was the entire universe, seen together or in its parts.

Over time, certain insightful philosophers tried to unify many aspects of human experience under general principles. Aristotle, for example, developed a comprehensive philosophy that began with a study of metaphysics (a study of being beyond the physical) and went on to include physics, ethics (governing social interactions), epistemology (science of how we know), and cosmology (worldview). This inclusion of both physical and metaphysical reality as objects of knowledge changed the interpretation of experience and scientific observation and analysis. Such was the business of systematic philosophy.

Our present culture also offers up cosmologies based on a certain set of premises, which often go unchallenged. Medicine bases itself on the premises of science, and life science has adopted an *a priori* empirical view of the world. Biology texts often begin by describing biology as the study of life, but then acknowledge that they cannot easily go further in defining it. They often assert that the human situation precludes our doing so. The inference is that the question "What is life?" is irrelevant. The prowess of physical medicine and scientific technology has discouraged us from questioning its underlying premise, that only events that are empirically measurable and observable have any worth. This extends to the universe, which covers more measurable and observable data than any individual can know. The apparent vastness of the universe is then taken as proof of the closure of this system. In this philosophy, or system of knowledge, it is presumed that only those things which can be scientifically proven exist. Such is the materialist philosophy of science.[2]

But others held a different view of things. From the beginning of recorded conscious thought, thinking people have challenged this materialist view of the world, intuitively recognizing that there is more to life and existence. Many writers have asserted, by weight of experience, that there is a transcendent level of reality to which tangible experience is related. In classic Greek times, Plato tried to reconcile these two views by postulating that the world of tangible experience was a reflection of another world, the world of ideas. We participate in the world of ideas whenever we engage in descriptive, categorical, abstract thinking. Thoughts and logic are as real as the physical objects they describe.

Furthermore, an object of our experience, such as a bird, depends for its reality on the extension of the idea of bird. Thus, birds all have something in common with the idea of bird in this ideal world created by our minds. What makes them alive is some sort of idea or activating principle coming from outside the individual.

Aristotle rejected this detached view of things. Instead he integrated the transcendent and tangible properties of each object in our experience by postulating that each thing has an essence—whatever marks it as belonging to a distinct categorical object—and an existence—its actual incidental being with particular individuating characteristics. Although they are logically distinct, essence and existence are inseparable in the individual thing. The same applies to the person. The life of an individual comes from a soul, which animates the material body. But, again, in the individual, body and soul are separable only from the standpoint of logic.[3]

## Philosophy and Bioscience

In looking at the question "What is life?" the materialist would argue that life is reflected in living things and that the individual is alive because of certain physical relationships on a gross, microscopic, and chemical level. In the opposing point of view—called vitalism—something is made alive by a "spark" or "element" from above or beyond its material constituents. This materialist/vitalist dichotomy in understanding the transcendent and immanent aspects of life, which began with Plato and Aristotle, has expressed itself differently in every age.

In the view of the sixteenth-century thinker Descartes, man is a material machine enlivened by a soul. Despite his adamant insistence that this distinction is intended only for the purposes of logic in understanding the various aspects of life, his view has historically been interpreted to mean a *dichotomy* between body and soul, the so-called "ghost in the machine" hypothesis. For a while this distinction seemed to satisfy both the materialists and the vitalists. However, during the nineteenth and early twentieth centuries, the materialist point of view took on a mechanistic approach, especially after the discovery of the microscope. Thus, while the microscope provided observable evidence of life on a smaller and smaller scale, it discovered no tiny soul within this complex matrix. For materialists, this was the proof they needed to once and for all quiet the vitalists, the implication being that, beyond the scope of our ability to see and measure, there is nothing else. If you cannot see it, it does not exist. Increasingly, the field of microbiology, amplified by many advances including those relating to genetics, seems to have defined the "machine" without needing another principle to define life.

Philosophers such as Henri Dreisch[4] and Henri Bergson[5] presented their ideas of *entelechy* and *élan vital* to complement the materialist's viewpoint. Each suggests a way to describe the "something else" in life that most people existentially appreciate. Although their ideas have not been well received by the scientific community, their legacy can be found in contemporary attitudes about the relationship between spirituality and medicine, nonlocalized healing effects, and subtle energy medicine.

## Osteopathy and the Materialist–Vitalist Dilemma

*Elements of Still's Synthesis*

Andrew Still, in his own reform of medicine, wanted the best of both philosophies, the materialist as well as the vitalist. He realized that medicinals, with their chemical basis, often failed. For those members of his family who were given medicine but nevertheless died, its premises were demonstrably false. Biological life could not be entirely explained in terms of chemistry, as the cutting edge of science in his day proposed.

Still, along with many others of his day, was taken by the ideas of Herbert Spencer, a systematic philosopher. Spencer argued that the entire universe follows the laws of Newtonian mechanics. In fact, the motion and interaction between objects even extends to the psychological, spiritual, and mental realms. Spencer saw creation, the making of living things, as the persistence of the creative idea. Persistence of ideas, or their reality, was a form of inertia and represented a force, just like the inertia of a physical object. Change between things, including relationships both physical and social, followed the laws of Newtonian physics, including the concepts of inertia, force, and mass:

> We come down finally to force, as the ultimate of ultimates. Though space, time, matter and motion are all apparently all necessary data of intelligence, yet a psychological analysis (here indicated only in rough outline) shows us that these are built up of, or abstracted from, experiences of force. Matter and motion, as we know them, are differently conditioned manifestations of force. Matter and motion are concretes built up from the contents of various mental relations.[6]

Elaborating on this thesis, Spencer reduced the chemical laws governing all of life to an interchange between attractive and repulsive forces. Furthermore, the operations of life—including thought, emotion, volition, and sensation—all required a transmission of energy that can be hypothetically proposed, but is more difficult to demonstrate.

Still himself was trying to bridge the apparent divide between physical anatomy and the spirit, trying to make his system comprehensive. He emphasized the mechanical viewpoint (more fundamental than the chemical viewpoint) by focusing on the interrelationship of structure and function and its importance to health. Yet, in order to explain the phenomenon of life—that special "something extra" of the vitalists—he introduced the concept of the Biogen.[7] Thus, the classic struggle to reconcile different aspects of our universal life experience is reflected in Still's intellectual odyssey:

> For thirty-five years I have observed man's body with the eyes of a mechanic so that I could behold and see the execution of the work for which it had been designed, and I have come to the following conclusion: The better I am acquainted with the parts and principles of this machine—man, the louder it speaks that from start to finish it is the work of some trustworthy architect; and all the mysteries concerning health disappear just as in proportion to man's acquaintance with this sacred product, its parts and principles, separate, united or in action.... I say yes, and treat the body as a machine should be treated by a mechanic.[8]

In this context, it is useful to revisit Still's inquiry into the nature of life:

> No one knows who the philosopher was that first asked the question, What is life? But all intelligent persons are interested in the solution to this problem, at least to know some tangible reason why it is called "life"; whether life is personal, or so arranged that it might be called an individualized principle of Nature.[9]

21

We see the form of each world, and call the united action biogenic life. All material bodies have life terrestrial and all space has life, ethereal or spiritual life. The two, when united, form man. Life terrestrial has motion and power; the celestial bodies have knowledge or wisdom. Biogen is the lives of the two in united action, that give motion and growth to all things. ... If a seed is planted in the earth and it obeys both the terrestrial and celestial forces, then the result is a tree. A man, biogenic force, means both lives in united action to construct all bodies in form, with wisdom to govern their actions. Thus Biogen or material life of the two obeys the wisdom of the celestial mind or life. The result is faultless perfection, because the earth-life shows in material forms the wisdom of the God of the celestial. Thus we say Biogen or dual life, that life means eternal reciprocity that permeates all nature.[10]

The majority of osteopaths have chosen selectively to attend to the first, or mechanical, aspect of Still's philosophy, avoiding the complexity of further thought. Attention is paid to models of treating the body from the material and mechanical points of view. Admittedly, Still's reflections on the transcendent aspect of life are often presented merely as allegories, dreams, or asides that represent Still's uneducated frontier style of expression, and are thereby easily dismissed. However, the problem of developing a model for dealing with what we euphemistically call the whole patient remains for our age, just as it did for Still's.

### Further Efforts at Synthesis

The mature clinician is aware that patients periodically present with evidence of causative factors that defy easy physical description. Intuitively, we reflect that our interior lives represent more than the pharmacological action of neurotransmitters or other psychoactive chemicals. The challenge of developing an osteopathic philosophy that is medically valid requires that we reformulate our experiences, as well as the experiences of those who came before us. This is part of the perennial struggle to refine, clarify, and make our understanding more complete. Osteopathic thinkers such as Sutherland, Becker, Fulford, Arbuckle, Barral, Upleger, and Jealous have all explored the mechanical as well as the nonmechanical dimensions of the patient.

This is the nature of the philosophical thinking that sensitized Sutherland to "dig on" and that motivated the young Fulford to reflect on the question "Who is my patient?" It should be remembered that Fulford was aware of Burr's L-field, and as a result, he may have been receptive to probing this question for several reasons. First, he may have concluded that there was sufficient data to bridge the apparent differences in the two philosophies. Second, perhaps Fulford felt that he had a sufficiently broad philosophic perspective in which to approach this area of the true nature of man and reality. Third, he was highly motivated to find a solution since this would help him discover novel, clinically relevant treatment procedures. He could legitimately ask, "Where in the context of this expanded definition of the person can I cooperatively intervene?"

Dr. Still insisted on understanding the body as it exists in Nature. This, in a sense, was a challenge to reexamine Nature, and the place of the human person in the universe—the essence of systematic philosophical investigation. Fulford saw this challenge as an integral part of medicine, not something that was alien to it.

## REFERENCES

1. Still AT. *Osteopathy Research and Practice.* Seattle: Eastland Press, 1992 (orig. 1910): 65.

2. Whitehead AN. *Science and the Modern World.* New York: New American Library, 1925: 20.

3. Montalenti G. "From Aristotle to Democritus via Darwin." In *Studies in the Philosophy of Biology.* Ayala F, Dobzhansky T (eds.) Berkeley: University of California Press, 1974: 21–24.

4. Dreisch H. *The History and Theory of Vitalism.* London: MacMillan and Co., 1914.

5. Bergson H. *Creative Evolution.* New York: Henry Holt, 1911.

6. Spencer H. *First Principles.* New York: A.L. Burt Publishing, 1880: 141.

7. Still AT. *The Philosophy and Mechanical Principles of Osteopathy.* Kirksville, MO: Osteopathic Enterprise, 1986 (orig. 1892, 1908): 249–51.

8. Still, *Osteopathy Research and Practice*, 12.

9. Still, *Philosophy and Mechanical Principles of Osteopathy*, 249.

10. Ibid., 251.

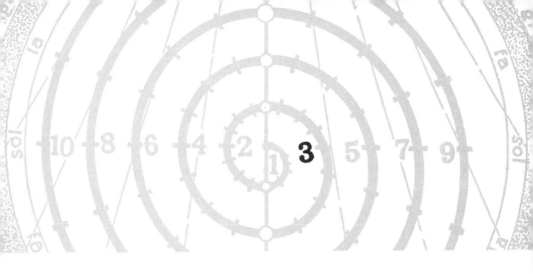

# This Doesn't Look Like Osteopathy!
## A Life's Journey

$\mathcal{A}$ll of us develop a unique practice style based on our own talents and life experience. Fulford's clinical approach, and the modalities that he used, were an expression of a long process of synthesis based on personal experience and inquiry. As noted in Appendix B, when Fulford was challenged with the accusation that his treatment did not "look like osteopathy," he defended his methods of diagnosis and treatment as an extension of osteopathic principles. In order to get people to keep looking further, Fulford would often emphasize the ways in which his methods contrasted with orthodox osteopathy. His intent, however, was only to challenge the osteopathic profession to reconsider its underlying premises and to deepen its understanding of people and life.

Fulford suggested including the energetic body in diagnosis and treatment, and considered this approach as a complement, albeit an essential one, to articular and fascial work. He wished no one ill, nor did he intend to give offense. Actually, he was a socially timid man caught in a bind between the burden of what he realized to be true and polite acquiescence to the consensus view. All of this makes more sense in the context of his personal and professional journeys.

## Personal Journey

Robert Fulford was born in 1905 to a professional family in Cincinnati, Ohio. His father, Alfred, was an attorney and his life was modestly comfortable. The family had some acreage and ran a small farm. Robert was sent out to work to build up his strength after a childhood bout with scarlet fever. He told tales of getting up early and milking, or carrying feed sacks. He associated this carrying, which he sometimes resented, with the recurrent left shoulder problem that bothered him through life.

Fulford had three sisters. One was injured in the head by a horseshoe that he had thrown in a game of horseshoes and died in childhood, never having fully recovered from the accident. The boy carried a burden of guilt into adulthood, but also resented the blame.

I include these personal details not as gossip, but to share that for each of us, our relationship to the patient and our mode of treatment involve working out our own place in the world. Fulford's identification with the conflicts of childhood was the basis for a strong and quick empathetic bond with many children who came to him as patients. The drive behind his attempts to heal and serve children, including grown-up children, came in part from the pain of his own conflicts as a child.

After Robert graduated from Ohio Northern University, a Presbyterian school, the family had plans to send him to medical school at the University of Cincinnati. Though spared the full brunt of the Great Depression of 1929, Robert was forced to defer his plans due to lack of funds. Instead, he took a job in the gas compression plant for Union Carbide, an experience that reinforced the work ethic begun at home. He also learned about the power of compressed force and the oscillatory motion related to the release of this force through control valves:

> This experience prepared me to understand the mechanical workings of the human body. Also how a minute change in structure would affect the function, the liquids and gases of the body.[1]

Later, in 1936, he reapplied to medical school after being told to make up an organic chemistry sequence. At the end of that summer, he would recount, he was called into the office of the dean of the medical school and told he had better consider becoming a dentist, not a physician. He left the meeting with a resolve to "show them." The following year he suffered an injury, and during the course of recovery, his desire to become a doctor resurfaced. A friend told him about the osteopathic profession. As a result, Fulford went to Kansas City, and, even though the term had started, he enrolled in the Kansas City School of Osteopathy and Surgery, now the University of Health Sciences. He graduated in 1941 and spent one year practicing in Rushville, Indiana, before returning to practice in downtown Cincinnati. During this time he married Glenna Graff, a young beauty, and began the family that included his two sons, Richard and David.

## Professional Journey

Beginning with the demands of early general practice during World War II, Fulford's professional life preempted his private life. Struggling to survive the work load of those days, when an osteopath was considered unfit for enlistment as a physician, but suited to care for the folks at home, Fulford would work twelve-to-fifteen-hour days, including night calls and home visits, until he fell asleep from exhaustion. It is no surprise that he searched for any treatment modality that would aid him in his work.[2]

### Experiments in Rhythmic Motion

Soon after graduation, Fulford heard of William Sutherland and the cranial approach to osteopathic treatment. In those days, Sutherland would train four students at a time in his office; then, after training was completed, would stay in touch with them. Fulford had the good fortune of being able to take the course.

Sutherland was a searcher for truth, and during this period he spent time with the philosopher, poet, and sculptor Walter Russell. Russell had an interest in physics and chemistry, which he considered to be an aspect of systematic philosophy. As noted in the previous chapter, he related all of this to a system of metaphysics and cosmology, branches of philosophy that are concerned with the concepts of who we are, how the world functions, and the creation of the universe. Russell's concepts complemented Sutherland's intuitions about the Tide, the rhythmic motion that describes important aspects of physiology.[3] Sutherland gave Russell the opportunity to apply his notions in the clinic. Together they conducted experiments, which unfortunately were not recorded. The young Fulford accompanied them and was quite excited about the implications of their joint work.

Fulford saw in the two men a commitment to the creative processes of the universe and of the individual. Observing their work, he developed a deeper appreciation for the notion of a connection between cause and effect, and for the universality of the law of motion, an idea inspired by the work of Herbert Spencer, who had also influenced Andrew Still. He witnessed Sutherland's struggle to integrate these new concepts into his work and felt that Sutherland backed off from doing so because of the political challenge of defending basic cranial concepts, such as central nervous system motility and the complex pattern of articular and membranous relationships.[4]

The concept of balance, and balanced rhythmic interchange, were key to Russell's cosmology. Fulford resolved to weave these new concepts into the work begun by Sutherland and Still. Eventually, this led Fulford to realize the importance of the intention or attitude of the physician, and of the rhythmic balance of forces in osteopathic theory and practice. In addition, this experience led Fulford to search for the right device to help recreate the "balanced rhythmic interchange" that Russell described as characteristic of healthy systems.[5] Fulford eventually settled on the percussion vibrator, described in Chapter 9.

*Effect of Pre- and Perinatal Trauma*

As a result of these ideas and influences, Fulford left The Cranial Academy for a while after Sutherland's death; he recognized these conflicts within himself and therefore thought that he was "not a faithful member" (see Appendix B). He spent time with Beryl Arbuckle, D.O., another maverick student of Sutherland's, who, as a pediatrician, had begun a program in Philadelphia for developmentally delayed children.

Having done hundreds of autopsies on infants, she recognized membrane patterns representing significant levels of dysfunction beyond those described by Still or Sutherland.[6]

These findings motivated Fulford to pursue the effects of pre- and perinatal trauma on infants and the application of this idea in the area of developmentally delayed children. Later he incorporated this as an important element in the history-taking of adults with complex or recalcitrant dysfunction.

### Respiration

Fulford learned to appreciate the multidimensional nature of respiration, largely as a result of meeting Edwin Dingle. While post-World War II families were discovering Disneyland, the Fulford family was visiting California to learn more about the works of Edwin Dingle, who had traveled Asia, and had opened the Church and Institute of Mental Physics in Los Angeles. Dingle introduced the Hindu tradition of prana and pranic breathing and their relevance to spirituality and health in a Western cultural context. This was the impetus Fulford needed to carry the significance of respiration beyond that which had been developed thus far in the cranial field. It introduced him to the idea that respiration has multiple levels of significance. It complemented the work of Arbuckle and Sutherland, and gave rise to the concepts of the Breath of Life and the First Breath, which will be discussed later.

### Energetic Life Force

As noted in Chapter 1, Fulford was greatly influenced by the Harvard neurophysiologist H.S. Burr, who, as a side project, had first measured the bioelectric field of trees, then of body tissues. Fulford was moved and galvanized by Burr's demonstrations. This became the foundation for his later pursuit of the connection between osteopathic therapeutic principles and the ethric body.

In his course on practice methods, Fulford would describe the history of this idea of an energetic force concomitant with life. In developing the idea, he included the Hindu concept of prana and the Chinese teachings on qi. He referred to the teaching of the Greek philosopher Pythagoras (c. 500 BC) on the "luminous body" and its physical manifestations, including its ability to aid in the recovery from illnesses. He cited the nineteenth-century works of Helmot, Messmer, and Von Reichenbach on biomagnetism. The latter conducted experiments with a field he called the "Odic force," and his model included a left and right polarity of the human body.[7] Early in the twentieth century William Kilmer, M.D., did comparable studies on the human energy field, and later the psychologist Wilhelm Reich used electronic and medical instrumentation to measure a pulsating energy, which he called the "orgone," that is shared by all life. In addition, he cited the work of Ravitz, Becker, and Russian scientists on the bioplasmic force. As Fulford pointed out:

> One of the important consequences of the field theory . . . is that the elec-
> tro-metric characteristics of the system in some way control the pattern of
> organization or, if you like, the design of the system.[8]

*Subtle Forces and the Nature of Life*

Fulford was very interested in Still's question about the nature of life and the role of subtle forces. Fulford's files were full of clippings, notes, and references regarding a wide variety of research into the theory of bio-physiologic forces, including endogenous fields, bioplasmic force, and psychosomatic connectivity, as well as their spiritual and/or cultural inter-connections. This was the milieu in which he practiced, integrating many of these concepts with his attentive, sensitive osteopathic palpatory find-ings, which, based on Still's conceptualization of the Triune Man, sought to diagnose and treat the whole person. Fulford believed that this was fully compatible with Sutherland's pursuit of subtle motion and forces within the framework of articular and membranous tissues—an expand-ed sense of the interrelationship of structure and function. The challenge was to keep one's feet on the ground and be scientifically critical while remaining open to exploring and treating in a venue of life that was not yet fully understood.

To that end, Fulford read the works of Still's contemporaries, including the previously-mentioned Karl Von Reichenbach and Wilhelm Reich, and their concepts of the Odic force and orgone.[9] These thinkers helped Fulford legitimize in his own mind the idea of a biodynamic force that is not generally accepted in contemporary medical physiology. In the early 1950s, he was reading Ralph Waldo Emerson, who had written about his belief in the pervasive rhythmic motion of creation and nature. Much of Fulford's thought revolved around a new view of the patient and of the cosmos. Emerson wrote philosophical poetry in a romantic vein reflecting on the place of man in nature. This helped Fulford see the whole person, as osteopaths have always claimed to do, in a larger context. Additionally, a neo-Emersonian, Newton Dillaway, described tone therapy, a way to use the rhythmic character of music to heal.[10] For Fulford this was yet another example of a practical application of the connection between rhythm and health. At the same time, Fulford was reading the works of Edward Bach[11] and integrating homeopathic remedies into his practice.

Later, in the 1970s, Fulford was exposed to the research of Robert Becker, M.D., an orthopedic surgeon working for the U.S. Veterans Administration. Becker had been experimenting with salamander limb regeneration, and, in a clever investigative sequence, determined that the form and extent of proper limb regeneration depended on a direct current field, which was an extension of the field of the body. Although his work led to the development of pulsed electrical charges to speed bone healing after fracture, the field theory aspect of his work was repressed.[12] This was one of the more substantive scientific contributions to Fulford's synthesis, further reinforcing the practical use of field theory.

Similarly, Fulford incorporated the work of Valerie Hunt, a neurophysiologist at UCLA, who wanted to measure what some called the human aura. Hunt, who began with the expectation of finding nothing of importance, discovered just the opposite: a scientifically measurable electromagnetic field that was significantly changed by the emotions of the subjects. She developed a protocol for measuring the human energy field, and her work led her to become a therapist in this area, leaving the field of dispassionate observation to others.[13]

Fulford saw in these ideas a neurological level of unification that substantiated some of the reflex associations he had been taught, and had experienced, in the body, especially those relating to trauma of various types. They validated his emphasis on the level of emotional involvement reflected in the solar plexus and its relationship to the diaphragm and respiration.

In the 1950s, around the time he picked up the percussion vibrator (see Chapter 9), Fulford met Randolph Stone. Stone was an osteopath who had traveled to Asia and returned with an integrated approach to osteopathy that included energetic input. He called his system Polarity Therapy, and taught that treatment should consist of proper polarity orientation and balancing of natural energy flow, and not the use of force, as in orthodox manipulative treatments. Inspired by meridian- and chakra-based models of the body from Asia, Stone saw dysfunction or ill health as resulting from a blockage of the natural flow and function of these energetic relationships in the body. An individual's growth and development on the physical, emotional, and spiritual levels was reflected in his or her symptomatology, and constituted the proper target for intervention. Stone saw this as an expansion of the osteopathic goal of restoring restricted motion: the healer's job was to facilitate the return of free flow.[14]

Fulford and Stone were impressed with each other, as evidenced by Stone's letters of appreciation and praise for Fulford's insights. Fulford, in turn, kept Stone's letters, and felt that Stone's success in healing was due to the powerful resonance of his voice. Stone's influence on Fulford will be further discussed in Chapter 4.

In the 1960s Fulford had contact with Marcel Vogel, another of those unexpected, but complementary, influences on Fulford's thought. Vogel reinforced Fulford's ideas about the interrelationship among the physical, emotional, and spiritual dimensions of the person. As suggested by Russell years before, they are related by the physics of the human organism; similarly, thought and intention—including the desire to serve in love—are forces with a physical dimension that can be used as part of the craft of healing. (Vogel's work is described further in our discussion of crystals in Chapter 9.)

In the 1970s, Fulford met and collaborated with Brenda Johnston, a British healer who came to the work through the efforts and teachings of Alice Bailey. Johnston's collaboration with Fulford reinforced his belief that the constitution of the individual, including the balance among the triune relationships, was paramount in determining the body's wellness. It also expanded his appreciation for the aphorism "Thoughts are things", a key idea of his in evaluating the source of dysfunction in socially-communicated sources of trauma. (Johnston's influence on Fulford is discussed further in Chapter 4.)

In 1979 Fulford moved to Tucson. He set up his practice and saw an increasing number of children, especially those with developmental delay. While in Arizona, he was sought out by Andrew Weil, M.D., which led to a documentary video[15] about Fulford and inclusion in Weil's book *Spontaneous Healing.*[16] Around 1986, at the encouragement of Gerry Slattery, D.O., Fulford and Slattery went on the road with a course to teach Fulford's use of the percussion vibrator. Shortly thereafter, he returned to a retirement community in Ohio with the intention of cutting back his practice. However, to the end he continued to see patients in his back sitting room that overlooked a cornfield.

As Fulford's eclectic interest in subtle and energetic healing became more widely known, his living room filled with material sent from contacts all over the world. To peruse the piles and shelves of materials was to enter a learning laboratory. In his later days he was significantly impressed by the neuropeptide work of Candice Pert. A pioneer in endorphin research, she discovered the system of the hormones of emotion, an ongoing research endeavor.[17] (The work and influence of Dr. Pert is discussed further in Chapter 5.) Fulford was also drawn to the work of Carolyn Myss, a psychic diagnostician who collaborated with Norman Shealey, a neurosurgeon who came to use complementary modes of wellness and pain management in his treatments. Myss's gift for psychic diagnosis, and Fulford's gift for alternative methods for controlling pain, led him to design his final treatment exhibition in which he treated the endocrine system of the body using a protocol called the "ring of fire",[18] discussed in Appendix B.

Fulford tried to reconcile the experiences of his intellectual journey with the state of contemporary osteopathic medicine. He welcomed students and other visitors to his home, and he visited nearby Ohio University College of Osteopathic Medicine on several occasions, as well as making frequent journeys to other osteopathic colleges. Fulford had long before returned to The Cranial Academy and published articles mostly relating to the treatment of children and the importance of birth, development, and correct cranial or total body function.[19] He had served as president of the group and supported the Academy until his death, trying to find a place there for the integration of his expanded osteopathic model. In 1992 he used his speech before the American Academy of Osteopathy to lay out his basic ideas. His final presentation, at The Cranial Academy Convention in Chicago in 1997, shortly before his death, was also a summation for him (see Appendices B & C).

Dr. Fulford participated as an active member of the Sutherland Cranial Teaching Foundation and the American Academy of Osteopathy, for whom he was a repeat convocation speaker. Underlying all of his presentations was the inclusion of the energetic body, and other forces, in the conceptualization of the patient.

Dr. Fulford continued to see patients, to read, and to think until his death on June 27, 1997.

REFERENCES

1. Robert Fulford's unpublished course materials.

2. The works of many of the individuals mentioned in this chapter are reviewed in more detail in Chapters 4 to 6.

3. Russell W. *The Universal One.* Waynesboro, VA: University of Science and Philosophy, 1926: 106, 197; *The Message of the Divine Iliad,* vol. 1. Waynesboro: University of Science and Philosophy, 1948: 74.

4. Sutherland WG. *Contributions of Thought.* Fort Worth, TX: The Sutherland Cranial Teaching Foundation, 1967: 132-33 (lecture delivered in 1948). See also Upledger JE, Vredevoogd J. *Craniosacral Therapy.* Chicago: Eastland Press, 1983: 1; Magoun HI. *Osteopathy in the Cranial Field,* 3d ed. Indianapolis, IN: The Cranial Academy, 1976: preface.

5. Russell, *Message of the Divine Iliad,* 74.

6. Arbuckle BE. *The Selected Writings of Beryl E. Arbuckle,* Camp Hill, PA: National Osteopathic Institute and Cerebral Palsy Foundation, 1977: 66.

7. Von Reichenbach K. *The Odic Force,* O'Byrne F (trans.) San Diego: The Book Tree, 2000; *Physico-Physiological Researches in the Dynamics of Magnetism, Electricity, Heat, Light, Crystallization, and Chemism as They Relate to Vital Force.* New York: J Redfield, Clinton-Hall, 1851.

8. Robert Fulford's personal notebooks.

9. Reich W. *Selected Writings: An Introduction to Orgonomy.* New York: Farrar, Straus, Giroux, 1973.

10. Dillaway N. *Consent.* Lee's Summit, MO: Utility Press, 1967.

11. Bach E. *Heal Thyself: An Explanation of the Real Cause and Cure of Disease.* London: C.W. Daniel Co., Ltd., 1931 (reprinted 1978).

12. Becker R. *The Body Electric: Electromagnetism and the Foundation of Life.* New York: Morrow, Williams and Co., 1987: 69.

13. Hunt V. *Infinite Mind: Science of the Human Vibration of Consciousness.* Malibu, CA: Malibu Publishing Co., 1989.

14. Stone R. *Polarity Therapy.* Sebastopol, CA: CRCS Publications, 1987 (orig. 1954).

15. Weil A. *Robert Fulford: An Osteopathic Alternative* (video). Tucson: University of Arizona, 1986.

16. Weil A. *Spontaneous Healing.* New York: Alfred Knopf, 1995: chapter 2.

17. Pert C. *Molecules of Emotion: Why You Feel the Way You Feel.* New York: Scribner, 1997.

18. Shealy N, Myss C. The ring of fire and DHEA: a theory for energetic restoration of adrenal reserves. *Subtle Energies* 6(2):167-75.

19. Some examples from *The Cranial Academy Newsletter:* "President's Message" (Winter 1974); "Physician, Treat Yourself" (Fall, 1979); "The Search for an Answer" (Fall 1979); "It's Written in the Bone" (Fall 1987); "The Primary Control" (Fall 1990); "Integration of Love with the Cranial Concept" (Fall 1998).

PART TWO

# Influences

"We see in man, as we comprehend it, the attributes of Deity. We see the results of the action of mind, therefore a representation of the Mind of minds. God is the Father of Osteopathy, and I am not ashamed of the child of His mind."

*—Andrew Taylor Still*

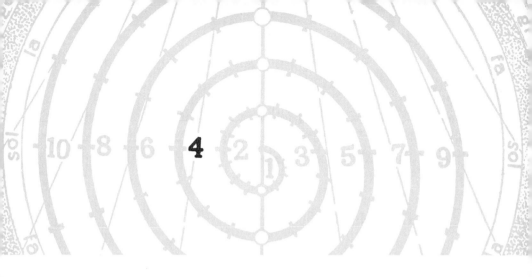

# From Philosophy to Methodology: The Constitution of Man

*A*s reflected in the philosophical debate in osteopathy between materialism and vitalism, discussed in Chapter 2, we make certain assumptions about the nature of the world and ourselves, which then become the premises for our queries. However, these premises are themselves subject to review and refinement.

Most of western medicine and science is based on a system of ideas derived from a Cartesian view of the world in which the body is regarded as an object and its rules of operation are based on the principles of Newtonian physics. Other cultures, and minorities in our own culture, have a different way of looking at the world and at the nature of the person. Andrew Still's premise of the Triune Man and the operating principles of biogenic life represent an attempt to reevaluate the conventional viewpoint. Still also suggested that God was the ultimate engineer, and that the osteopath was the ideal mechanic. This was his effort to find a home for the transcendent aspect of life under the umbrella of the Newtonian worldview.

As discussed in Chapter 3, through a series of influences beginning with Burr and his L-field, Fulford reformulated the osteopathic approach to the whole person based upon a different way of viewing the patient and of viewing life. Most notable among these influences were Walter Russell, Randolph Stone, and Brenda Johnston. It is worthwhile exploring the thoughts of these individuals further in order to more fully understand Fulford's synthesis of ideas, which guided his clinical practice on a daily basis.

## Walter Russell (1871–1963)

*Community of Thinkers*

Earlier we mentioned the meeting of Fulford, Sutherland, and Russell. Russell had been a writer and sculptor, a consummate man of the arts. Together with his wife Lao, he had formed a community of individuals with common interests, preaching a new world order based on a certain systematic philosophy in the classical tradition. Perhaps through his sense of proportion as an aspect of beauty, Russell had adopted a philosophy along the lines of Pythagorus, in which rhythm and harmony are not just pleasant and entertaining, but are the organizational principles of the universe itself. All creation is a complex of interrelated, periodic motion. In his quest to shape this into a systematic philosophy, Russell extended the concept of "balanced rhythmic interchange" into the areas of chemistry (elaborating upon the periodic table of known elements and predicting new ones),[1] economics, and the social order.[2] He was, no doubt, pleased to be able to extend it into physical medicine through his dialogue with William Sutherland.

*Rhythmic Forms and Patterns*

Perhaps because he was an artist, Russell expressed his view of the universe and of man through diagrams. In his later years, his writings took on the form of aphorisms or syllogisms. It is an unusual style for us to read today.[3] He gathered together a circle of intellectuals including Oliver Wendell Holmes, Walt Whitman, Mark Twain, Andrew Carnegie, and John Burroughs. They called themselves the Twilight Club, which was based on the belief that, unless some new direction were taken, they were reflecting on the twilight of civilization. The Russells founded a teaching center, the University of Science and Philosophy, in Waynesboro, Virginia that survives today and is still true to its original mission: a community involved in world change through the intelligent application of logically ordered, loving concern about world problems.

Russell's principal concept was that there is a divinely ordained intellectual order to the universe which underlies the physical forms we experience. Nature, ourselves included, can be better understood by paying attention to these intrinsic relationships which are expressed as rhythmically patterned motions. Similar to the order of creation described in Christian scriptures at the beginning of the Gospel of St. John, he developed an emanation theory of cosmology in which the Creative Force was a word or idea which was disseminated through the cosmos as light. In his theory, light is used to describe discernible "influences" which are not limited by Newtonian physics. He intimated that these influences were compatible with the dual wave–particle nature of light and the convertibility of matter and energy. In addition to this cosmology, Russell proposed a new physics and theory of understanding of the true nature of the individual.[4]

This dissemination of energy and form is responsible for all aspects of our experience, and physical matter simply reflects a step-down form of higher levels of creative vibratory energy. The characteristics of individual elements in the periodic table demonstrate this relationship between matter and form, he said, and because of his faith in the rules of rhythmic relationships, Russell postulated the existence of unknown elements based on the properties of those that were known. Some of these elements have, in fact, subsequently been discovered (Figs. 4-1 & 4-2).

One of the concepts that makes Russell's ideas attractive to osteopathic thinkers is the importance he attached to motion. He viewed all motion as an expression of attraction or repulsion between opposites:

> Modern science is perfectly familiar with the oscillatory motion of electromagnetic force, and also with the fact that opposed oscillations are opposed forces.

41

Attraction and repulsion are the apparent effects of the opposites of motion.

One is an effect of revolution, the other of rotation. … One is an effect of gravitation, the other of radiation.… One is an effect of contraction, the other of expansion.… One is an effect of inhalation, the other of exhalation.[5]

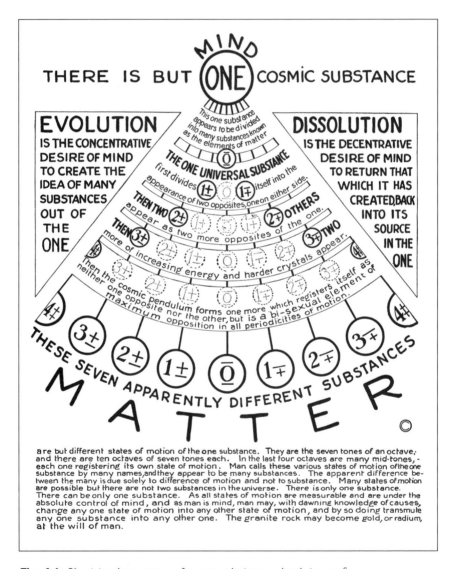

**Fig. 4-1** Chart tracing source of many substances back to one[6]

In an elaborate expansion of his ideas, Russell, in *The Universal One*, described the relationship of apparent opposites and their creative electromagnetic significance as complementary spiral cones. The apices of the spiral cones are the focal points of the high potential of their system, the high point of evolution or development. This is Russell's way of express-

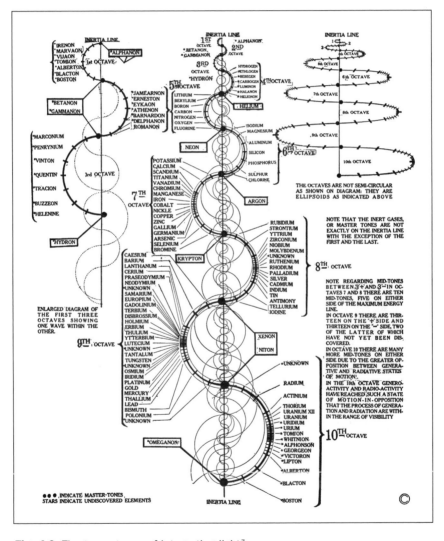

**Fig. 4-2** The ten octaves of integrating light[7]

ing a scheme to describe the relationship between the material and the immaterial aspects of reality as distinct but inseparable, using concepts drawn from chemistry and physics. Materiality and immateriality reflect different series in the progression of order. Within each series, there is a repeating pattern of order, referred to as a spiral. Just as chemical elements repeat in series dependent on the activity of their subatomic particles, so too is spirituality ordered in a similar pattern of energetics. Likewise physiology or physical well-being. Both the material and the spiritual dimensions of our world are striving toward completion—the apex of each spiral of development—by reunification with the source of creative energy, the Mind, or divine creative intelligence. Disease, unhappiness, and interpersonal strife all reflect a resistance to cooperate in this spiral of development toward completeness.

Russell's system represents an emanation theory of philosophy, of which there have been many in human history. (In emanation theories, a succession of beings arise from a single source.) Russell was ambitious in attempting to incorporate modern science and psychology into his schema. He represented in Fulford's time what Herbert Spencer had been in Still's time.

For the individual, the goal of a happy and successful life is to partic-ipate in this progression of growth in the spiritual and material dimen-sions. Both dimensions are governed by the laws of rhythmic motion. On the physical level it includes our physiological motion as well as our res-piration and locomotion. On the spiritual and emotional planes it includes love and meditative consciousness, which reflects openness to the creative power of Love and Light. All of these relationships share an energetic dimension, which is cyclic, periodic, or vibratory.

Russell's writing style is aphoristic and dense, and it is difficult to find specific ideas with clinical application. However, Fulford used his ideas to validate his own belief in the vibratory characteristics of well-being, and to identify the cause of pain or illness in the interruption of this vibrato-ry motion pattern in the individual. It also complemented Fulford's belief in the functional significance of the L-field or life field. Finally, it made him appreciate the commonality among physical, emotional, and spiritu-al trauma.

In Russell's and Fulford's worldview, acquiescence to this process of individual development is the source of health, and resistance to it, or to be obstructed in the process, leads to disease. Pain and dysfunction are but incidental signals. Disease, therefore, reflects inappropriate relationships, including that of the energetic state. This imbalance is manifested in symptoms, and on a more significant level, in developmental arrest. Vibrations are not limited to the physical plane, but also involve our psychological and spiritual aspects. Each represents a level of activity and a source of potential resonance. Therefore, health must take into account the emotional and spiritual disposition of the person, including their relationship to the Creator. In this cosmology, love is a force capable of causing physical change, and is a part of healthy living and healing.

Russell drew upon the emerging field of quantum physics and the discussion about the dual nature of light, and, as befitting a sculptor, made appropriate modifications to his philosophy and to his theories of psychology and physiology. Ideas and thoughts were likewise active principles. One's thoughts, or those of another making a suggestion to you, could distract from your growth process. Thus, the words and behavior of others can also contribute to our developmental arrest.

In Chapter 3 we mentioned the influence of Herbert Spencer on Andrew Still.[8] Coincidentally, Russell's own system began as a reflection on the thought of Spencer. One can see, then, how a man like Sutherland, or Fulford, would find philosophical compatibility with Russell's writings and would try to adapt some of his ideas about mind, matter, and motion to the clinic. This would be in keeping with Still's challenge to clinical medicine. We can see in Russell's philosophy the seeds for reinforcing such Sutherland concepts as the bent twig, the universal importance of rhythmic motion, the physiologic and ontological significance of respiratory motion, the implication in this motion of the action of the Creator, and the application of these ideas to the resolution of physical symptoms. Indeed, an astute French osteopath, Francois Bel, recently traced the influence of Russell on Sutherland's thought.[9]

Russell's system is an expansive one which requires extensive personal reading to digest. A synopsis of his thought can be found in a book by Glen Clark, *The Man Who Tapped the Secrets of the Universe*.[10]

Here are several passages from *The Universal One*[11] containing ideas that were later integrated into the thought of Robert Fulford:

The physical is a reflection of a higher process.

All reality is in rhythmic flux between polar opposites—the rhythmic balanced interchange.

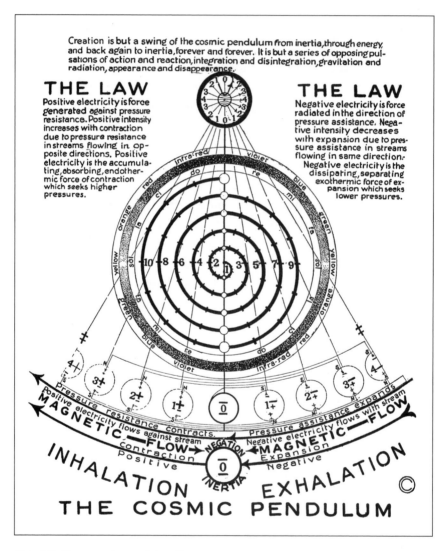

**Fig. 4-3** The cosmic pendulum[12]

Creation is ordered as serial 'step-downs' of higher energy states.

Light is the highest known element.

The Material body is a 'near-crystallization' form of energy.

Life belongs in principle to motion.

All motion is periodic and evolutionary.

The Universe breathes, in inhalation and exhalation.

All motion is equilibrium between motion in opposition and motion in inertia.

All that appearance which man calls matter is motion in opposition.

Motion in inertia is equally electric and magnetic.

All motion is oscillatory, as a pulsating inbreathing and outbreathing, as an inhalation and an exhalation, which is characteristic of all motion whether it is units, or systems, or mass.

Matter is Light gravitationally assembled into the appearance of form and radically disassembled into the disappearance of form.

Fulford considered Russell to be one of the greatest thinkers he had ever encountered. He read him and encouraged others to do the same. This influence is apparent in many of Fulford's ideas, which he reiterated over and over again in his teaching career:

- Thoughts are things.

- Trauma is a disruption of patterns of motion.

- Personal development is an aspect of motion and somatic dysfunction.

- The role of the healer is to remove blockage to energy flow.

- The mind of the patient and of the healer are important parts of the healing process.

Evidence of Russell's influence can be found as well in Fulford's course notes. Here, for example, are Fulford's notes on the concept of the balanced rhythmic interchange:

Balanced Rhythmic Interchange between pairs of opposites.... Balance is the principle of unity. In it lies the stability which lies cause.... Balanced Interchange, equal giving between all moving parts of unbalanced opposites.... Rhythmic, Balanced Interchange is the principle of continuity of effect. Continues. Repetition.

Material things follow the pattern of energy.... Energy follows the pattern of thought.... Thought follows Universal Manifestation.... Universal Manifestation follows the nature of Being.

Below these notes he drew a tetrahedron, at the angles of which are the words Spirit, Body, Mind, and Love. Under this was the inscription:

One with the universe, a tetrahedron.

Tetrahedron is the dimension of Water Molecule; the human body is 70% water; water is the tree of life.

## Randolph Stone (1890–1981)

*The Wireless Anatomy of Man*

Randolph Stone was schooled in the chiropractic and osteopathic approaches to health. Nevertheless, he felt compelled to pursue further the questions of Who is man? How is he made? and Which interventions facilitate health? These questions led him to India, where for years he studied those aspects of traditional spirituality that were applicable to health. He became aware of the need to integrate personal development with the sense of a level of organization that was higher than the mere physical.

Like Russell, Stone was drawn to the notion of understanding physical health in terms of a subtler dimension, an electromagnetic one that was an extension of thought or spiritual forces. Like Russell, he saw all of creation as an expression of resonant energetic patterns. However, unlike Russell, who saw all this motion as a balance between polar opposites, Stone saw the world in triadic relationships. In Stone's system, the point of balance was a nameable entity (neutral), as were the polar opposites (positive and negative). The concept was expressed in a system called Polarity Therapy that relied on what Stone called the "wireless anatomy of man." He chose this term because he realized that he was describing a human bio-electrical function without reference to the nervous system.[13]

In a series of books elaborating the relationships and principles that were key to his understanding of the nature of life, death, and disease, Stone integrated what he learned from the traditional eastern point of view with modern western anatomy and physiology. These books contain many drawings to illustrate his thoughts, diagnostic approach, and treatment methods. This enormous task resulted in an integration of the eastern appreciation for extra-material forces with contemporary healing arts. From this expanded view of the nature of man came a treatment approach with a different focus:

> Polarity is the principle of the triune essence and energy in all created things. It is the energy in motion, expression, and in sensation.
>
> In this atomic age of science, we realize that matter itself is but a mass of spinning energy particles which appear as solid substance. In reality they exist as such only because of a constant flow of energy between all parts and portions. As soon as that circuit is interrupted, changes begin to appear which, in the human body, are interpreted as pain or disease.[14]

Compare this passage with a statement made in an address by Fulford at the 1992 Convocation of the American Academy of Osteopathy:

> The human body is composed of complex streams of moving energy. When these energy streams become blocked or constricted, we lose the physical, emotional, and mental fluidity potentially available to us. If the blockage lasts long enough, the result is pain, discomfort, illness, and distress.[15]

As previously noted, according to Stone the organization of every level of life was dependent on the correct relationships between polar opposites and their balance point. Stone took this idea from the Hindu theme of balance among three complementary forces or gunas: satva (neuter), rajas (positive), and tamas (negative). Each of these forces has different phenomena and qualities (Table 4-1).

**Table 4-1** Matrix of the main correspondences of the polar opposites and their balance points

| POSITIVE | NEUTRAL | NEGATIVE |
| --- | --- | --- |
| Soul | Mind | Body |
| Causal body | Ethric/emotional body | Physical body |
| Source | Action | Crystallization |
| Supraconscious | Conscious | Subconscious |

An analysis of this matrix for ordering reality shows that the constitution of the person is more complex than just their physical body, motion characteristics, or symptoms. Stone took the osteopathic concept of the interrelationship of structure and function and applied it to this more complex system. To begin with, his concept of the body parallels Russell's in its attention to the energetic characteristics of motion. Furthermore, he envisioned the energetic activity at the body surface to be divided into left and right fields of activity. Energy flow on the right side is from head to toe anteriorly, and continues from foot to head posteriorly. On the left side of the body, there is a complementary flow in the opposite direction (Figs. 4-4 & 4-5).

According to this system, the head and foot are balanced between opposite polarities and the midsection contains the neutral point. A subset of this arrangement includes a similar pattern at each joint, with a positive pole proximally, negative pole distally, and a composite neutral balance point when the tissue is healthy.[16]

In addition, there is an internal core energy flow of intersecting positive and negative channels that crosses at a system of energy centers. These correspond to the Hindu chakras, or energy wheels. Interestingly, this relationship is also reflected in the pattern depicted in the Greek and Roman classic symbol of the caduceus, the snake on the staff, which has been incorporated into the medical insignia. These energy centers have anatomic and physiologic significance, partly corresponding to conventional anatomic and physiologic function. More importantly, they represent key sites in the energy body worthy of evaluation for proper function in both diagnosis and treatment (Figs. 4-6 & 4-7).

Besides the system of major centers aligned along the central axis, there are a number of minor centers, including those in the hands and feet. The polarity of these minor centers is important in defining Stone's approach to palpation and treatment.

Unlike Russell, Stone was a clinician, and his theoretical model was

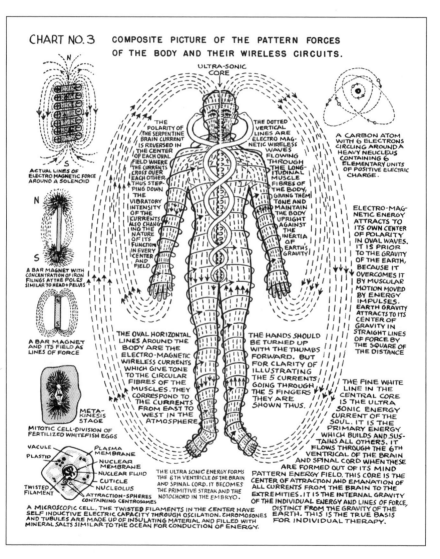

**Fig. 4-4** The pattern forces of the body and their wireless circuits[17]

therefore accompanied by a wealth of detail concerning practical applications. Fulford was greatly influenced by Stone's ideas concerning diagnostic and treatment methods, both of which are partly described below. These ideas are reflected in Fulford's methodology.

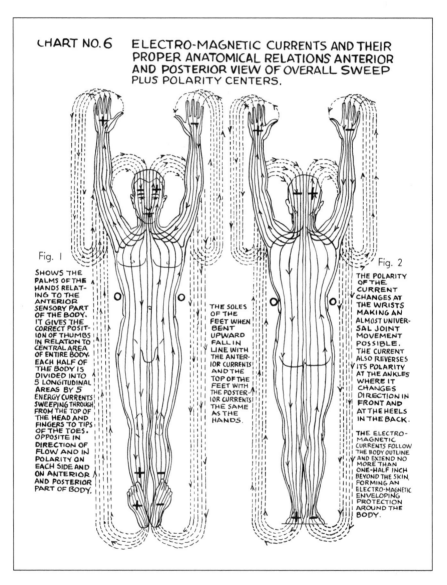

**Fig. 4-5** Electro-magnetic currents and polarity centers[18]

In general, the pathways proposed by Stone are electromagnetic in nature, and their organization in the body does not follow the nerve pathways. Instead, they follow electromagnetic field dynamics, hence the name "wireless anatomy of man." Stone's model is compatible with myofascial theory,[19] but hysteresis is viewed in Stone's model as the result of not just tension, but more precisely of tension plus alteration of field potential. Stone was an osteopath trained in an era when the focus was on

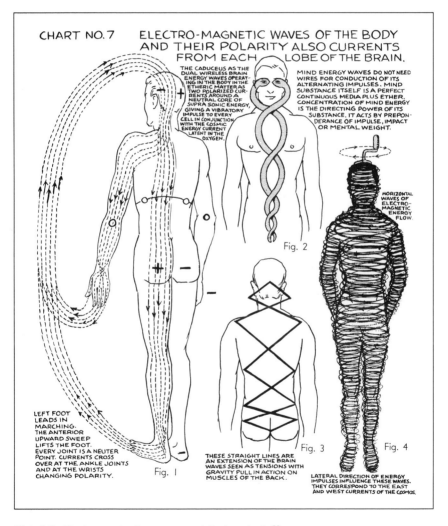

**Fig. 4-6** Electro-magnetic waves and their polarity[20]

articular integrity. For him, however, articular mobility resulted from field fluidity, not disrupted joint mechanics.

In terms of diagnosis and treatment, this relationship is important because proper function—or the proper electromagnetic field underlying the visible physical structure—relies on the healer working with the elec-

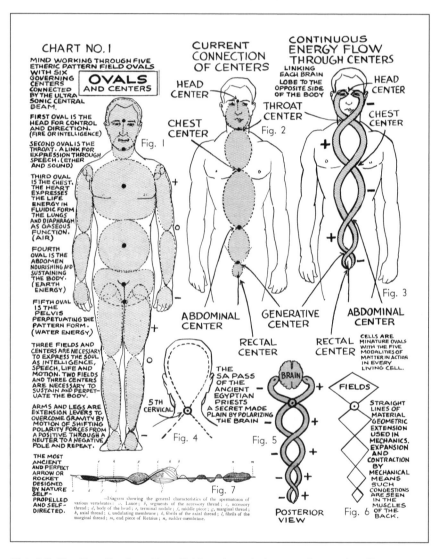

**Fig. 4-7** The five etheric pattern field ovals and six governing centers[21]

tromagnetic interactions, rather than applying mechanical force. In the fields of chiropractic and osteopathy, only a minority of practitioners, such as William Sutherland, Charlotte Weaver, and Charles Naylor, relied on subtle relationships and forces in their treatments.

The hands can be used to sense both the field dynamics and the mechanical tissue state. For example, to sense the field, the practitioner approaches the patient's right side with his or her left hand to create a complementary, and therefore neutral, interaction as a base line. Variation from the normal base state is then palpable as subtle perturbations in the field. Additionally, the energetic charge of the hand as a minor center serves as the basis for sensing imbalances between the patient's major centers.

Stone recommended treating by improving the balance at the centers; the practitioner's own "field contact" is used to oppose any unbalanced charge. In other words, if, for example, there is an overabundance of positive energy on the right side of the body creating a physical problem in the thoracic spine, the practitioner will position the patient in such a way as to oppose that flow by the proper placement of his or her right hand. Stone's books are full of illustrative drawings that surpass any verbal description (see Figs. 4-8 & 4-9).

In this approach, pain is evidence of a disruption in the flow of energy. As with any other osteopathic method, the key to a successful treatment is determining the underlying cause. Stone looked for this in the energetic body. He maintained that this blockage was palpable if one directed one's attention to discovering it. In addition, he incorporated classic studies of the spine and posture into his theory and developed a force diagram for weight distribution of the spine that seems to parallel the work of the early twentieth-century English osteopath Littlejohn.[22, 23]

A derivative concept of this organizational scheme is the role of the companion vertebrae in health and disease. This concept is of clinical significance since the spine is a unit, and often a dysfunctional vertebra requires treatment of its pair complement in order to be successful. Pairing is ordered in a mirror image pattern around C3 and L3 as the primary pair (Fig. 4-10).

CHART NO.18.   MEASURING THE LEGS FOR COMPARATIVE LENGTH
TO DETERMINE THE SIDE OF THE MOST CONTRACTED ELECTRO
MAGNETIC CIRCUIT WHICH IS ONE DEFINITE MEASURE OF
IMBALANCE, DISTINCT FROM GRAVITY.

GRASPING THE SIDE OF EACH FOOT
WITH A GENTLE BUT FIRM TOUCH
EVERT THEM TO STRAIGHTEN THE
HEELS AND BRING THEM TOGETHER
SLOWLY WITH THE
BIG TOE JOINTS
MATCHING. THIS GIVES
THE OVERALL PICTURE
OF THE LENGTH AT THE
BOTTOM OF THE HEELS.
CHART THE SHORT
LEG ONLY

THE ELECTRO MAGNETIC FIELD ON EACH
SIDE OF THE BODY IS THE OVERALL
CURRENT WHICH IS RESPONSIBLE
FOR MORE TENSION ON ONE SIDE
OF THE BODY THAN THE OTHER.
SEE CHART 8 –FIG. 4.

Fig. 1

Fig. 2

IN ILLNESS, THE BODY IS OUT OF BALANCE; THERE IS MORE
TENSION AND OBSTRUCTION ON ONE SIDE AND THIS IS THE INHERENT
WEAK SIDE FROM BIRTH, THAT SHOWS UP IN EVERY ILLNESS.

ANOTHER CONTACT
FOR MEASURING
THE LEGS IS SHOWN
HERE WITH THE HANDS
UNDER THE HEELS AND
ANKLES – BENDING THE
HEELS OUT TO STRAIGHTEN
THEM – THEN BRING
THEM TOGETHER AND
LOOK FOR COMPARISON
AT THE HEELS FOR THE
LENGTH OF LEGS. THE
SHORT LEG IS THE
FACTOR.

KEEPING THE
ELECTRO MAGNETIC
FIELDS IN BALANCE
WOULD BE A FINE
HEALTH MEASURE.
BALANCE OF ENERGY
CURRENTS MUST BE
RESTORED IN EVERY
SICKNESS BEFORE
HEALTH CAN BE
REALIZED.

WHEN THE SHORT LEG
HAS BECOME LONG AND
STAYS LONG, IT INDICATES
THAT THE TENSE
MAGNETIC FIELD ON
THAT SIDE HAS RESPONDED
AND NORMAL REPAIR
CURRENTS ARE, AT WORK.
THE PATIENTS IMPROVE-
MENT WILL VERIFY IT.

Fig. 3

Fig. 4

EVEN LEGS
INDICATE
IMPROVEMENT
AND ARE
CONSIDERED
NORMAL.

Fig. 5

Fig. 6

Fig. 7

SHOWING THE LEFT
LEG SHORT.

A SIMILAR CONTACT IS TAKEN WITH THE PATIENT FACE DOWN. EVERT THE
FEET, SO THERE IS A STRAIGHT LINE DOWN THE CENTER OF EACH LEG TO
THE HEEL AND COMPARE THEM. MEASUREMENT DIFFERS SLIGHTLY IN THIS
POSITION FROM THE FRONT MEASUREMENT.

**Fig. 4-8** Measuring legs to determine side with most contracted electromagnetic circuit[24]

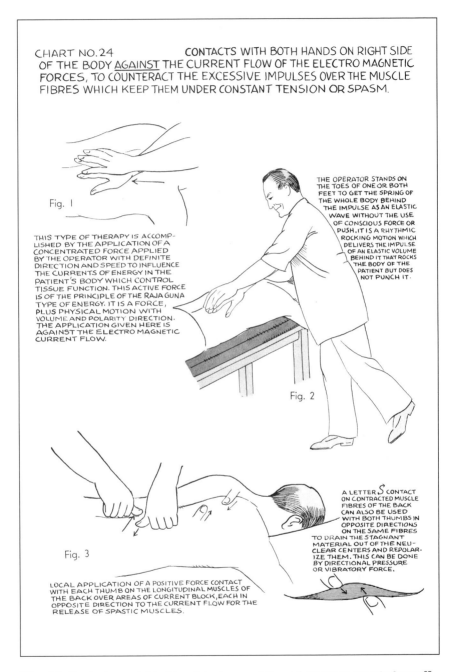

CHART NO. 24       CONTACTS WITH BOTH HANDS ON RIGHT SIDE OF THE BODY <u>AGAINST</u> THE CURRENT FLOW OF THE ELECTRO MAGNETIC FORCES, TO COUNTERACT THE EXCESSIVE IMPULSES OVER THE MUSCLE FIBRES WHICH KEEP THEM UNDER CONSTANT TENSION OR SPASM.

Fig. 1

THIS TYPE OF THERAPY IS ACCOMPLISHED BY THE APPLICATION OF A CONCENTRATED FORCE APPLIED BY THE OPERATOR WITH DEFINITE DIRECTION AND SPEED TO INFLUENCE THE CURRENTS OF ENERGY IN THE PATIENT'S BODY WHICH CONTROL TISSUE FUNCTION. THIS ACTIVE FORCE IS OF THE PRINCIPLE OF THE RAJA GUNA TYPE OF ENERGY. IT IS A FORCE, PLUS PHYSICAL MOTION WITH VOLUME AND POLARITY DIRECTION. THE APPLICATION GIVEN HERE IS AGAINST THE ELECTRO MAGNETIC CURRENT FLOW.

THE OPERATOR STANDS ON THE TOES OF ONE OR BOTH FEET TO GET THE SPRING OF THE WHOLE BODY BEHIND THE IMPULSE AS AN ELASTIC WAVE WITHOUT THE USE OF CONSCIOUS FORCE OR PUSH. IT IS A RHYTHMIC ROCKING MOTION WHICH DELIVERS THE IMPULSE OF AN ELASTIC VOLUME BEHIND IT THAT ROCKS THE BODY OF THE PATIENT BUT DOES NOT PUNCH IT.

Fig. 2

A LETTER $S$ CONTACT ON CONTRACTED MUSCLE FIBRES OF THE BACK CAN ALSO BE USED WITH BOTH THUMBS IN OPPOSITE DIRECTIONS ON THE SAME FIBRES TO DRAIN THE STAGNANT MATERIAL OUT OF THE NEUCLEAR CENTERS AND REPOLARIZE THEM. THIS CAN BE DONE BY DIRECTIONAL PRESSURE OR VIBRATORY FORCE.

Fig. 3

LOCAL APPLICATION OF A POSITIVE FORCE CONTACT WITH EACH THUMB ON THE LONGITUDINAL MUSCLES OF THE BACK OVER AREAS OF CURRENT BLOCK, EACH IN OPPOSITE DIRECTION TO THE CURRENT FLOW FOR THE RELEASE OF SPASTIC MUSCLES.

**Fig. 4-9** Contacts on right side against current flow of electro-magnetic forces[25]

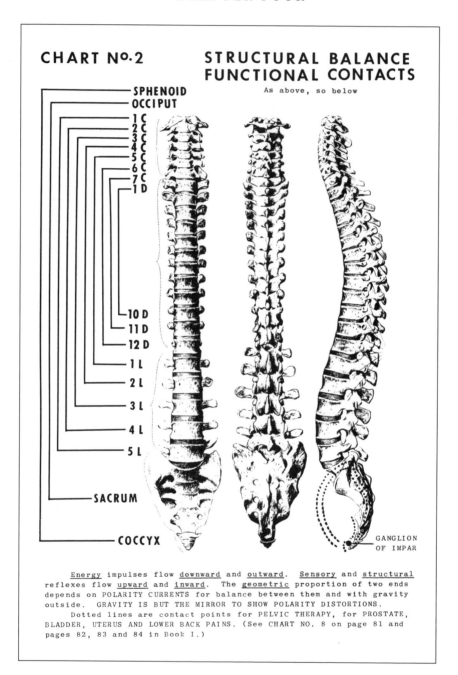

CHART Nº.2

STRUCTURAL BALANCE
FUNCTIONAL CONTACTS

As above, so below

SPHENOID
OCCIPUT
1 C
2 C
3 C
4 C
5 C
6 C
7 C
1 D

10 D
11 D
12 D
1 L
2 L
3 L
4 L
5 L

SACRUM

COCCYX

GANGLION
OF IMPAR

Energy impulses flow downward and outward. Sensory and structural reflexes flow upward and inward. The geometric proportion of two ends depends on POLARITY CURRENTS for balance between them and with gravity outside. GRAVITY IS BUT THE MIRROR TO SHOW POLARITY DISTORTIONS.

Dotted lines are contact points for PELVIC THERAPY, for PROSTATE, BLADDER, UTERUS AND LOWER BACK PAINS. (See CHART NO. 8 on page 81 and pages 82, 83 and 84 in Book I.)

**Fig. 4-10** Structural balance functional contacts[26]

In this arrangement, the pairs consist of:

- C1 and L5
- C2 and L4
- C3 and L3
- C4 and L2
- C5 and L1

The following passages from *Polarity Therapy* encapsulate Stone's interpretation of osteopathic technique:

> The body moves by action of leverage through its joints. It overcomes gravity through mechanical leverages. Is it not energy, from the body's own Central Sun of energy within itself? Hence it is a reaction from within to the great without, as the Life Breath of motion which moves through all cells, like the wind through a forest.
>
> Each joint has a relationship to each other joint in the unity of energy flow of graceful motion. The ankles, the knees, and the hip joints and the shoulder joints are important factors in the Polarity Action as extension levers of motion, with polarity actions *on other ethers and fields in the body*. And because they are moved by a unit of energy current though them, energy circuits in the body can be reached through their corresponding area of relationship, as illustrated in my books.
>
> Our aim is to balance the nervous systems in their bipolar effects with the circulation of the flow of 'prana' in the body. As these two contacts are held, changes will take place.
>
> Skill in treating plus understanding of the energy fields in the body are the key factors.[27]

In addition to facilitating present maximal function, Stone looked at the state of personal evolution of the patient as part of the diagnosis, goal setting, and treatment. This reinforced the idea of Walter Russell's that personal health includes unrestrained personal development.

Fulford attended teaching sessions by Stone in Chicago in the early 1960s.[28] Their correspondence reflects the mutual respect and sense of identification between the two men. Stone's method of working provided Fulford with many of the practical points that he would later integrate into his manual treatment techniques, as well as those utilizing the percussion vibrator. Key concepts that he adopted from Stone include the polarity of the hand contact, attention to the field for restriction, and the idea of the energetic life breath. The umbilical area was deemed highly important because of its embryological significance, as well as its involvement with the body's energy centers, the midpoint of a polar body. The idea of gently rocking a body part in both diagnosis and treatment is another idea derived from Stone.

## Brenda Johnston (b. 1916)

### Background

As noted in Chapter 3, the healing methods of Brenda Johnston served to consolidate and add detail and nuance to Fulford's methods. He corresponded with and then visited this British healer (which included some cooperative healing sessions), who had been introduced to energetic healing through Alice Bailey. Johnston, in turn, has passed down her approach in this country to Barbara Briner, D.O., among others.

Alice Bailey was the daughter of a Christian minister serving in India. As a young adult, she was involved in programs of Christian service and ministry to the British colonial troops. Without solicitation or formal contact with the Theosophical Society or other spiritual organizations, she received the aid of a Himalayan wise man who appeared in her life at times of need and led her on a path to a more universalist expansion of her former beliefs. She continued her life of service, and was progressively given insight into the nature of the world and man's place in it from the point of view of Hindu thought.[29]

### Thoughts are Things

Brenda Johnston was taught by Alice Bailey. As with Randolph Stone, in her treatments Johnston believed in the importance of joining hand contact with intention. The intention is a potential link with the person, providing an avenue for helping the individual progress in his or her development. This progress comes from integrating the multiple levels of the person's being, including the body, and through union with higher powers. Our present world can be seen as one level in a hierarchical unfolding of existence, much like the emanation theory of Russell's. Viewed from the level of the individual, the organization pattern is one in which the physical body is the lowest level of participation in the life of the individual (recall Stone's approach). Symptoms in the physical body are rarely the cause of a problem; more likely than not, symptoms reflect an energetic predisposition to dysfunction in the *etheric body*, which is the subtler aspect of the physical body. Johnston described the etheric body as the term used in the ancient wisdom literature that corresponds to the electromagnetic or bioplasmic body being investigated by a handful of scientists:

> The etheric body, which we call it here, is composed of fine interlocking lines of energy, in constant circulation, emanating from one or more of the seven planes, or areas of consciousness, of our planetary life. It also channels the lines of light or force from our own subtler vehicles, our mental and emotional aspects, and all these are poured from the etheric body into the physical counterpart.[30]

This etheric body is palpable six to eight inches from the surface of the physical body. The physical body is important, but does not fully explain the identity of the person, the nature of his or her experience, or the true nature of the trauma that induced the symptoms. The extended definition of the person includes the mental and emotional bodies, which in turn are in union with the triad of Love, Will, and Higher Mind, all of which transcend the individual. This union is mediated by the soul.

Suffice it to say that physical symptoms and disease are reflections of a much larger process. They can reflect an appropriate, though incomplete, developmental stage in the individual's evolution, or they can reflect a growth crisis, necessitating a choice or intervention. In treating the physical body, it takes some discernment to distinguish among the possibilities and to determine which circumstance is currently dominant in the patient. Simply put, success in treatment and success in symptom improvement are not equivalent. The healer's job is to become attuned to the higher level of existence, then join with the patient and facilitate the "next best step." This may or may not result in the immediate relief of symptoms.

In addition, successful healing incorporates the idea of union with one's own soul. The soul, or higher mind

> overshadows the personality and maintains a direct connection with the man by means of a thread of energy called the 'thread soul', during the entire span of earth-life. The Soul is group-conscious and is one with all other souls.
>
> If we think on the Christ, merge thought and feeling in the Christ, com-

mune with Christ and blend our minds with the Mind of Christ, a new
rhythm will be silently but surely imposed upon every phase of our personal
activity.[31]

Treatment is thus seen as "interventional" attunement of the practitioner,
the patient, and the higher mind. It proceeds by an ontological, intentional entrainment of energized states drawing the patient to a higher
level of function through the agency of the healer. Specific palpable tar-
gets, reflected in the main energy centers of the body individually or in
interrelated patterns, are treated with light contact and the intention to
heal. In this, we see the roots of Fulford's commitment to the use of an
invocation, and the importance he attached to intention. It also recalls
Sutherland's admonition to "stay close to your maker." An extension of
this is the method of diagnosing by intuition.

This is not to say that the physical body, in their view, is bereft of
value. The physical body is an important source of information. Energy is
palpable for specific organs and energy centers, and the spine, as the axial
representation of many of these energy centers, is important in diagnosis.
In addition to the physical disposition of individual vertebral segments,
the energetic character of the spine is assessed by attending to its energetic characteristic by using the hand's own centers during palpation.

As was the case with Stone and others who influenced Fulford, Johnston
reiterated the fact that man is in the adolescent stage of a profound developmental process. The main thrust of this process is the appreciation of
one's unity with all creation through the development of one's soul, which
is a participation in life in its totality. The physical body is one aspect of
the vehicle in which we travel during this process, and its state, or symptoms, are but a shadow of this deeper developmental process. With this
emphasis, Johnston does not discuss the specifics of physical diagnosis,
but she goes into much more detail about the comportment, on many levels, of the healer. Here is her description of proper palpation:

> The hands are related to the reception, distribution and manipulation of
> energy. Energy as we know follows thought, directed from the Ajna or crown
> (of head) center and the two hands make up a triangle round which the
> thought directed energy can flow. In healing, Man is using himself like a
> Transformer, receiving energy from the spiritual Source, passing it through
> him, and transmitting it as force through his hands and centers.[32]

This theme of triangular relationships is repeated in several different ways, as in

- Using the hands and Ajna
- Emphasizing the relationship of the healer, patient, and Source
- Occasionally using two healers plus the patient.

The task of healing, rather than being concerned with symptoms, is to check the centers for balance, look for imbalance or altered vibration, and intentionally balance the centers. All of this occurs in the context of attuning oneself to the needs of the Soul, seeking assistance for the higher self, and linking the healer and patient with the Soul, the only "healer within the form."

We can see in this the derivation or reinforcement of Fulford's frequent comment that "thoughts are things" and the need to diagnose and treat through the etheric (or "ethric") body. We can also see the origin of Fulford's idea that energy blockages reflect developmental delay, and the importance he attached to emotional blockages.

### REFERENCES

1. Russell W. *The Universal One*. Waynesboro, VA: University of Science and Philosophy, 1974 (orig. 1926): 4, 12.

2. Russell W. *The Message of the Divine Iliad*, vol 2. Waynesboro, VA: University of Science and Philosophy, 1948: 60-103.

3. This passage from page 27 of *The Universal One* is typical:

   > *Consider an idea of Mind, whether that of individual man or the Universal One.*
   > *Man thinks idea.*
   > *Thinking is the force of motion.*
   > *All motion is expressed in waves.*
   > *All waves of motion are both male and female.*
   > *All motion is oscillatory action and reaction.*
   > *Action is male. Reaction is female.*
   > *All idea is registered in light as an appearance of the form of idea.*
   > *Form of substance is electromagnetic.*

4. Russell, *The Universal One*, 1-20.

5. Ibid.

6. Ibid., p. 9.

7. Ibid., p. 13.

8. Trowbridge C. *Andrew Taylor Still: 1828–1917*. Kirksville, MO: The Thomas Jefferson University Press, 1991: 117.

9. Bel F. *William Garner Sutherland át-il été influencé par Walter Russell*. *Apostil* 2000; 6:14–22.

10. Clark G. *The Man Who Tapped the Secrets of the Universe*. Waynesboro, VA: Walter Russell Foundation, 1956.

11. Russell, *The Universal One*.

12. Ibid., p. 11.

13. Stone R. *Polarity Therapy*, vols. 1 and 2. Sebastopol, CA: CRCS Publications, 1987 (orig. 1954).

14. Stone, *Polarity Therapy*, vol. 1: 11.

15. Based on author's notes of Robert Fulford's statement to the 1992 Convocation of the American Academy of Osteopathy.

16. Stone, *Polarity Therapy*, vol. 1, book 2: 13.

17. Ibid., p. 10.

18. Ibid., p. 13.

19. Friedman H, Gilliar W, Glassman J. *Myofascial and Fascial-Ligamentous Approaches in Osteopathic Manipulative Medicine*. San Francisco: San Francisco International Manual Medicine Society, 2000: 6.

20. Stone, *Polarity Therapy*, vol. 1, book 2: 14.

21. Ibid., p. 8.

22. Littlejohn JM. *The Fundamentals of Osteopathic Technique*. Maidstone, England: Institute of Classical Osteopathy, 1975: 120–24.

23. Campbell C, ed. *The Osteopathic Technique of John Wernham* (video with diagrams). Maidstone, England: Institute of Classical Osteopathy, 1996.

24. Stone, *Polarity Therapy*, vol. 1, book 2: 25.

25. Ibid., p. 31.

26. Ibid., vol. 2, book 5: 15.

27. Ibid., vol. 1, book 3: 5-24.

28. Personal communication from Robert Fulford, 1993.

29. Bailey A. *Esoteric Healing*. New York: Lucis Publishing Company, 1991.

30. Johnston B. *New Age Healing*. Havant, England: self-published, 1978: 6.

31. Ibid.

32. Ibid.

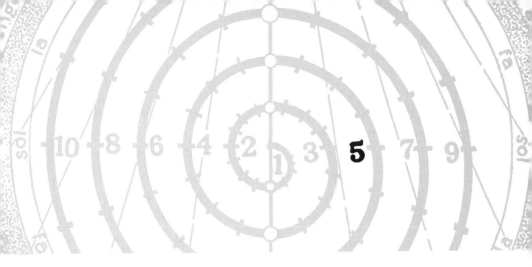

# 5

# Scientific Validation of the Human Energy Field: Fulford's Contemporaries

### Robert Becker, M.D. (b. 1923)

*The Fascia as Piezoelectric Tissue*[1]

We have previously mentioned the importance to Fulford of the work of H.S. Burr and his early electronic measurement of biodynamic fields in nature. This work was also of interest to Robert Becker, M.D., an orthopedic surgeon and researcher who worked for years under the auspices of the United States Veterans Administration. Becker revisited many of the same issues in his quest to investigate the body's capacity and mechanisms for healing. His work sheds light on the issue of the electromagnetic aspect of the body.

Initially intrigued by limb regeneration in the salamander model, Becker saw parallels in the healing process—especially of fractures—in other animals and in younger children. Limb regeneration and fracture healing involve the reproduction of appropriate materials as well as the restoration of bodily form. Early in his studies, Becker validated the observation that trauma to a limb induced a current of injury, with a positive charge in the limb relative to the trunk, and that in the early stages there is a conversion to a negative charge. He noted that, in humans and salamanders, the extremities have a negative baseline while the trunk and head have a positive baseline. He also noted a native direct current that was distributed through the nervous system of an organism; this current was distinct from the alternating current-like axonal propagation of depolarization of the action potential. The extent and strength of the DC charge could be altered by cutting a nerve, administering anesthesia, or otherwise manipulating the state of consciousness of the organism.

The end, practical result of Becker's work was the clinical application of electric current to facilitate fracture healing, especially those fractures that did not join correctly in the early stages. However, he was quick to point out that separating this application from an understanding of the basic electromagnetic character of the body and its function was inappropriate.

Becker's synopsis of the experimental evidence in *The Body Electric*[2] notes that two key issues that are often unappreciated in the initiation of healing are the electromagnetic impetus for the repair, and the quality of the regenerative forces, both of which are related to the nature of the electromagnetic field described above. Some of these findings had been adequately covered elsewhere in the study of genetic expression, growth factors, and the differentiation of mature tissue to pleuripotent cells with subsequent differentiation into the required cell lines for tissue repair. However, the question of the *form* of the organization seemed to Becker to be dependent on some non-depolarizing aspect of neural function. He went on to hypothesize and test the theory that the distribution of this formative field in the organism appeared to be that of a semiconductor undergoing conduction and rectification, and allowing biochemically active electrons to travel freely in the field.[3] Under these conditions the body functioned like an ordered crystal. This complements the conventional paradigm of biochemical interaction.

Fulford viewed Becker's findings as a more contemporary validation of the early work of Burr, which Becker also cited. It galvanized Fulford's belief that an individual's energy field is important to the body's structure and function. This opened the door to a reconceptualization of the unity of the body through the redefinition of the fascia, often thought of as simply structural connective tissue, as piezoelectric tissue. When he introduced the concept of an energy field to scientifically trained physicians, Fulford first discussed the work of Becker, encouraging them to read *The Body Electric.*

## Valerie Hunt, Ph.D. (b. 1916)

*Further Measurements of the Energy Field*

Valerie Hunt and Robert Fulford were both interested in the human energy field. Hunt, originally a skeptical UCLA neurophysiologist, experienced a career crisis in the course of her effort to study the relationship among thoughts, emotions, and the physical body. After being challenged to do so by her students, she measured the neuromuscular activity related to emotion and found that this led to an investigation of auras and altered states of consciousness and their role in healing. While she had an early personal experience that was compatible with these nontraditional ideas, her adult persona—that of a professional, critically rigorous scientist—prevented her from accepting and validating her childhood psychic adventures.

Eventually, she performed EMG (electromyography) on dancers as they experienced altered states of consciousness and was confronted with a variety of EMG anomalies which were at variance with the view of classical neurophysiologists. Furthermore, she found meaningful relationships in the baseline, that part of the signal of lower amplitude usually filtered out as noise. In this millivolt range, she measured fluctuations that correlated to changes in the auras as reported by auric readers. Using NASA's discarded telemetric recording devices to analyze the power-density and frequency spectrograms, she demonstrated a field that oscillated at frequencies of 250 to over 20,000 Hz. Manipulating this field in a MU room (an electromagnetically isolated space), she showed that the field was reactive to changes in the electromagnetic environment, and that these changes registered as subjective emotional changes in the patient, including fatigue, stress, and anxiety. She summarized her conclusions:

Although composed of the same electrons as inert substances, the human energy field absorbs and throws off energy dynamically. It interacts with and influences other matter, whereas fields associated with inert matter react passively. Again, there have been many names associated with this known energy, chi, life force, prana, odic force, and aura.[4]

Hunt drew parallels between the frequency and voltage patterns generated by her data and those chaos attractor functions found in analyses of brain waves, weather data, and other natural phenomena. It would appear that these attractor patterns represent the body's own conductive process and that they have consequences for the individual's health.[5]

The question, however, is whether this contrasts with basic cell theory, the basis for most of biochemical interaction in the body. Hunt's argument echoed that of Becker:

Orthopedist Robert Becker's studies and mine give the most extensive evidence that healing occurs through changes in the electromagnetic field. At the cellular level of molecular circuits, there are endless electro-windings as well as microtubular array of collagen, that is, connective tissue, the support structure of all tissue. At every level through the body, from the cell, to molecule, to atom, there are structural evidences of the intrinsic electromagnetism of life. The whole body oscillates. It has even been speculated that the non-resistive superconductive circuits at the molecular level intimately connect life on a global basis.[6]

Hands-on and healing by one's presence emphasize the transaction between two people, each with an intent—one to become well and the other to serve as a catalyst. I believe the best healer does not attempt to heal; that belongs to the healee. But rather the healer intends to present a positive, enlightened presence to manifest a strong, radiant, complete field and encourage the ill field to change.[7]

Hunt cited supporting data regarding integration of physiology, consciousness, and emotional processes. This led her to a career change where she used this research as a basis for biofeedback in individuals with psychological and emotional problems. She is now translating as much of her work as possible into a more easily understandable treatment modality.

Fulford viewed this work, rooted in the rigor of legitimate science, as substantiating Burr's L-Field. In some of his introductory courses he would demonstrate the field, perhaps extending six feet from the body, through the use of a simple dowsing apparatus such as a metal coat hanger wire. He also saw the frequency of vibration of the individual as reflective of their state of personal evolution. He would say that a more evolved individual would vibrate at 700 or 800 Hz, the average individual under 200 Hz. He would reflect that, in the 1930s and 40s, when there was more of a spiritual or ethical undercurrrent to society, people vibrated at a higher frequency and were generally easier to treat.

Fulford saw the connection of this work to Russell and Stone, and to Johnston's concept of an etheric body that is important to the development of the individual. With regard to treatment theory and methods, he saw Hunt's work as paralleling his own and validating his efforts to change the symptoms of an individual by intentional manipulation of the field. In his advanced percussion vibrator courses, he recommended that the participants read Hunt's work *Infinite Mind.*

## Candice Pert, Ph.D. (b. 1946 )

*Molecular Biochemistry*

The word *consilience* describes the act of concurring, or the coincidence of findings, with the implication that this was not the original intent or expectation.[8] Fulford's reading area was (not surprisingly) stacked with periodicals from the Institute of Noetic Science, the International Society for the Study of Subtle Energy and Energy Medicine, and the published thoughts of many writers who were pursuing the new paradigm of the social and hard sciences linking health and consciousness. In these we can see a trend.

In addition, his reading table held a copy of Candice Pert's *Molecules of Emotion.*[9] We had both read and discussed this book. Dr. Pert wrote that, as a precocious graduate student in a high-powered neurophysiology laboratory, she had been involved with the discovery of the opiate receptors. She said that in 1972 her colleagues had a difficult time accepting the fact and significance of the discovery. The fact that natural endorphins interact with the same receptors as exogenous opiates is now widely accepted, but the significance of this discovery is still evolving.

As her physiochemical work continued, it became apparent that the internal biochemical communicative milieu of the body is not only one of basic body regulation, but also involves a neural integration process tied to a psychoemotional integration process. She later described one aspect of her work as identifying the *molecules of emotion*, since changes in emotions resulted in changes in neuropeptide balance and vice versa. These molecules of emotion vary with an individual's social interactions and other personal experiences, some of which can be traumatic in nature, and can, in turn, contribute to the individual's mood, behavior, and physical well-being. These relationships are therefore also important for clinicians.

Pert's subsequent work included the identification and mapping of a great number of neuropeptides in the body. Such biocompounds were previously thought to be closely associated only with synaptic activity, within microns of their release site in the peripheral and central nervous systems. By contrast, chemicals acting at a distance were usually classified as hormones. Pert's mapping clearly showed that this division between neurotransmitters and hormones was not so distinct, and that peptides of neural—even brain—origin were active at many sites throughout the body. Not only were these compounds associated with visceral organs, they were also associated with cells of the immune system. Monocytes had receptors for contact with neuropeptides; what is more, they sequestered and released these as part of the cascade of events involved in the immune response.

Pert further pointed out that visceral-active peptides, such as cholecystochinin, had visceral-mediating and central nervous system effects. The body, in effect, was a neurochemically interbalanced network.

In support of her work, Pert cited Ed Bloch's writings from the early 1980s. Bloch conceived of a system known as the psychoneuroimmune complex. Pert's work began as an elaboration of the specific players in this system. The unifying concept that emerged was that neural substances previously known to mediate or to be evoked by an emotional response were shown to be involved in the body's fight against foreign antigens.

Pert's work was also cited by Valerie Hunt, since the qualitative and quantitative aspects of ligand binding are compatible with the properties of energy fields, that is, the molecular interactions occurring with behavior and mood states reflect populations of receptors and ligands acting in phasic patterns.[10] These, in turn, produce measurable gross changes in the function of the organism, possibly through the generation of a field.

Additionally, since neuropeptides, thoughts, and the individual's physical state were linked, Pert's synthesis was a potentially titratable and measurable corollary to Fulford's belief that "thoughts are things." Thoughts have physical consequences when, for example, emotionally charged words and actions are used; they can create in oneself and in others, through the language of shared experiences, a change in physical function. If these patterns form loop interactions and feedback loop interactions, a new state, once initiated, could continue indefinitely until something occurred to break the loop. Threatening encounters are emotionally charged, and trauma, either physical or perceived, can harm the organism.

Fulford accepted this as evidence from a scientific source for the substantiation of the reciprocal relationship between body and mind, emotion and thought. What is more, it occurred on a molecular level, which had its own level of electrochemical interaction. Pert had a limited understanding of the musculoskeletal system and the potential for integrating her findings at that level. Fulford, however, made the connection that emotions, through respiration, controlled the bodily form.

In fact, Fulford's way of describing the somatic effect of trauma included the shock of trauma, which involved the physical arrest of respiration from residual diaphragmatic tension. This phenomenon, however, was linked to the emotional event associated with the physical trauma (if present). This is discussed in Chapters 6, 7, and 8. It should, nonetheless, be noted here that it is a key idea.

As will be further elaborated in later chapters, the physical area beneath the lower ribs in the epigastrium—the solar plexus—was called the *visceral brain* by Fulford. Besides constituting the autonomic plexus associated with the abdominal viscera, the solar plexus corresponds to the third chakra in the Vedantic vision of the body, as reflected in Stone and Johnston's approaches.

Fulford's affinity for the description of the body as an energy process was consistent with Pert's model of a receptor-ligand network in the sense that both reflected a subtle, nonmechanical balancing of self-regulating systems. In addition, both were physical in nature, but included emotional and cognitive inputs and effects. Fulford saw this type of balancing of ideas across disciplines as supportive of his approach to the body, and superior to a purely mechanical or hydraulic model.

## REFERENCES

1. Piezoelectricity is the observed flow of electrons in a material initiated by physical stress or pressure.

2. Becker RO, *The Body Electric: Electromagnetism and the Foundation of Life*. New York: William Morrow, 1985: 95-102.

3. Ibid., 93-9.

4. Hunt V. *Infinite Mind: Science of the Human Vibration of Consciousness*. Malibu, CA: Malibu Publishing Co., 1989: 20.

5. Ibid., 330-33.

6. Ibid., 240.

7. Ibid., 265.

8. Wilson EO. *Consilience, The Unity of Knowledge*. New York: Knopf, 1998.

9. Pert C. *Molecules of Emotion: Why You Feel the Way You Feel*. New York: Scribner, 1997: 183.

10. Hunt, *Infinite Mind*, 249-52.

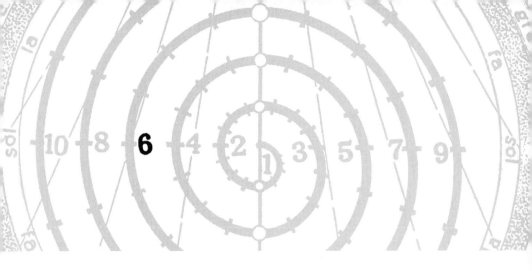

# 6

# The Significance of Respiration, Including the First Breath

## Breath of Life

*A*s previously noted, Fulford, like Sutherland and Still before him, attributed a special significance to respiration. A creative, eclectic assimilator of ideas, Fulford's thinking in this area built upon that of his predecessors. Yet the concept of the First Breath, with its special clinical applications, reflects many of Fulford's original ideas.

### Sutherland's Understanding

Sutherland believed that the respiratory cycle affected the potency of vitality on several levels. In *The Cranial Bowl* he described respiration as a profound and fundamental aspect of motion, the indigenous motility of the body, coextensive with life.[1] He asserted the primacy of the cranial respiratory mechanism, and the secondary importance of diaphragmatic respiration.[2] Only in extended footnotes did he postulate the brain's spontaneous movement. In comments long overlooked, he cited Dr. Dwight Kenney in an address to the Minnesota Osteopathic Society:

> Kenney called attention to the molecular electromagnetic potency of the blood corpuscles as the impelling power to the circulating blood, rather than

the muscle activity of the heart; and that the cerebrospinal fluid circulates under the same law. The amount and efficiency of this electromagnetic power is naturally attendant upon our reserve of vitality.[3]

In another note he described his personal experiments in concentrating on stilling the endogenous motility and resultant "fluid wave" of his own primary respiratory mechanism.[4] However, beyond these notes, the balance of the book emphasized the articular mechanics, membranous tension, and fluid dynamics of cranial movement. The emphasis throughout the book is on motion.

Sutherland also noted the profound effect of motion restriction on an individual's development. In the well-accepted elaboration of Sutherland's system, Harold Magoun discussed the primary cause of birth-associated respiratory suppression, anesthesia administered to the mother:

> Generally speaking, failure to breathe effectively is due to drug depression or anoxia or mechanical trauma which has locked the cranial mechanism. It is in this field that the cranial concept is most useful.[5]

In this expression of Sutherland's thought, the respiratory "mechanism," and the response of the body, are dealt with primarily from the mechanical point of view.

### Fulford's Understanding

Primed with many of Still's mechanical analogies and Sutherland's focus on the aspect of respiration joining vitality, rhythmic motion, and oxygenation, Fulford probed deeper, teasing out other functional implications of respiration. Communication among Fulford, Sutherland, and Russell generated the idea that rhythmic motion reflected the motion of life that was transmitted from the Creator as thought and love. In Sutherland's clinical applications of the cranial rhythm concept, Fulford saw the particular relevance of this idea to palpable physiology. Arbuckle's expansion of Sutherland's thought in exploring the connection between physical health and stress-inducing agents during the birth process confirmed in

Fulford the importance of the birth moment to the continuing health of the individual.[6]

Russell led Fulford to see the interconnections of being, moving, and breathing in the creative act. These had psychological, spiritual, and physiologic implications. The quality of life of the person was tempered by the quality of all these experiential elements.

So, for Fulford, the palpable quality of respiration ("The Breath") in symptomatic patients represented the composite of influences on the individual of their physical and psychological health and trauma history from prebirth to the present. Again, the best medium for appreciating the quality of an individual's vitality was the energetic body; the physical body and its diaphragmatic respiratory pattern were helpful, but were not as sensitive or deeply revealing.

Not surprisingly, in his course description on the importance of the breath, Fulford cited the constancy and the vital necessity of breathing, as well as its association with thought. He noted that, unlike other autonomic vital functions, this process can be subject to voluntary control:

> Due to this double nature, breathing can be made the mediator between mind and body, or the means of our conscious participation in the most vital and universal functions of our psychosomatic organism. Thus the conscious control of the breath affects the electrical polarity of the brain and our biophysical luminescence.[7]

Fulford would often assert that each new breath initiated a new thought, or a "turn" in a current thought. He connected breathing with the cerebrospinal fluid: "The 'primary conductor' for the life energy in our body is the cerebrospinal fluid. The cerebrospinal fluid is ionized by breathing exercises."[8]

Fulford also frequently cited Still's mention of the vital capacity of the cerebrospinal fluid to irrigate the "withered fields," so often quoted to us by Sutherland and his other students. Fulford's insistence on nasal breathing was partially based on the proximity of the olfactory bulbs in the cribiform plate of the ethmoid bones to the flow of oxygen in the nasal passages.

# First Breath

"As a man breathes, so he is."[9]

With this aphorism, Dr. Fulford laid the connection to the importance of the First Breath, involved in both our individual existence and our continuing vital capacity. Fulford held that the observable pattern or quality of the patient's breath was partly a shadow of the quality of the actual first breath of the individual.

In teaching his courses, Fulford would present the form of the fetal skeleton in utero and an artist's rendition of the baby moving through the birth canal (Fig. 6-1), which showed the birth presentation with the left side of the occiput engaging the barriers. Sutherland had described the importance of all this for mobility of the cranial base,[10] and Arbuckle had indicated that the variable pattern of anterior stress bands reflected the imprinting in the membranes of intrauterine stress.[11]

Fulford recommended inclusion of the Leboyer method of childbirth to allow the delivered infant to lie on the abdomen of the mother prior to cutting the umbilical cord.[12] The purpose of the Leboyer method was to moderate the abruptness of change in circulatory patterns. In this pose, the inhalation phase of the First Breath would expand the cranial bones in a more relaxed manner and initiate a more complete expansion of the whole body, resulting in life-long consequences for the health of the individual.

The exhalation phase of the First Breath was the baby's first cry. Fulford cited the work of Truby in Sweden, who conducted a longitudinal study of 15000 infants in which he compared the sonographic recording of the first cry to their first seven years of development.[13] Truby found that from the form and intensity of the cries he could predict the personality, weaknesses, and relative health of the children. For Fulford, there remained the question of what would have happened if the children in the study with the weaker cries had been rescued.

In his presentations, Fulford would add other references, including the works of Chamberlain, Verny, and Diamond, to describe the significance

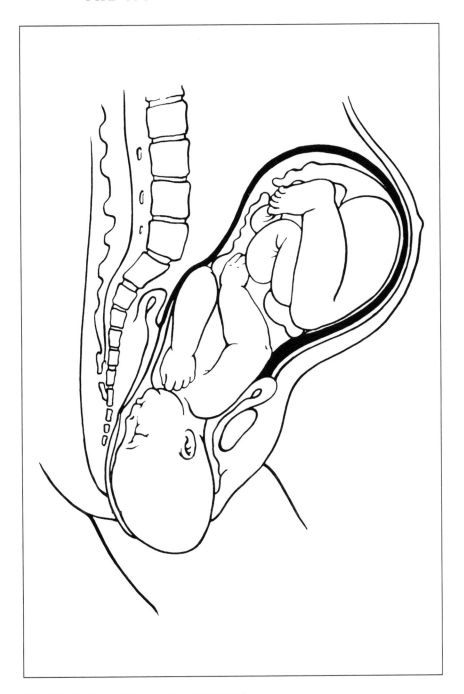

**Fig. 6-1** Position of baby in the birth canal.

of pre- and perinatal life on the infants' functional status. Thomas Verny, M.D., summarized two decades of medical research on the baby's capacity to pay attention, to feel, and to remember.[14] As a psychiatrist, he was mostly concerned with the psychological well-being of the children and their subsequent lives as adults. The intimate bond of mother with child made her an ideal conduit for many of these experiences. He cited evidence for physical responses in a child, such as the heartbeat, to thoughts of the mother. Patterns of thought or attitude could strongly affect the health and vitality of the newborn, and memories were shared. Stress, including social stress, precipitated fear in the fetus and avoidance behavior, such as kicking.[15] Although Dr. Verny's focus was on personality disorders and growth delay from the psychological point of view, his summary of the research on prebirth and perinatal experience confirmed Fulford's belief in the significance of this period in the health of the child and the adult.

David Chamberlain's book *Babies Remember Birth*[16] paralleled this point of view from a psychologist's perspective. He found that hypnotized adults and young children had memories of the prebirth period and the birth process. This work was based largely on the memories of individuals during interviews and therapy sessions.

John Diamond is a psychologist and past president of the International Academy of Preventive Medicine. His work as a whole reflects a commitment to the idea that the body and psyche progress in parallel during the developmental process of the individual. He places special significance on the birth process in diagnosis and in treatment. In his copy of Diamond's book *Life Energy*,[17] Fulford highlighted those pages involving "birth trauma." Diamond related the deeper issues of fear, hate, and envy that some claim accompany the infant's leaving the comfort of the womb. He believed that the birth event was socially conditioned and that a fearful, anesthetized woman dropping a baby in an alien and sterile environment may induce fear and other negative emotions in the baby. The alternative of a more natural childbirth, for example, following the methods of Leboyer, was preferred:

If a baby can be born without this deep fear, there will be no death instinct, there will be no hatred; he will grow up in a beautiful, loving household, a high-thymus household. His experience of negative psychopathological states will be minimal. He will be creative. He will evolve.[18]

Diamond reflected on the benefits of cranial osteopathy as a complement to a Leboyer method-based birth: "With the Leboyer birth, for example, the first breath opens up all these suture bones and opens up the whole body so that the baby's normal development can take place."

Diamond proposed a method for testing the individual's sense of security as reflected in the memory of the birth experience. Using the paradigm of muscle strength testing from behavioral kinesiology, he assessed the patient's response to several stimuli that provoked a birth memory. Most, due to the trauma of the birth process in our culture, showed a negative "comfort test." Diamond then proposed a therapeutic intervention in the form of role playing to reprogram the emotional response to the birth experience. In this form of kinesiologic testing, muscle tone is tested in a relaxed, unprovoked state, using the opponens pollicis muscle. Upon presentation of a test stimulus, repeat testing of the muscle demonstrates a positive or negative effect of the stimulus on the individual, as reflected in the muscle's strength or weakness. Diamond noted that: "The comfort test problem relates to the baby's first breaths. Thus it is not surprising that the specific primary meridian of involvement is the lung meridian, which is called the first meridian."[19]

Fulford met and corresponded with Diamond. Fulford grasped the significance of reprogramming the birth experience to reverse subsequent developmental arrest underlying symptoms, even in adults. He incorporated these ideas into his multidimensional approach for treating symptomatic adults and children by using a method that was simultaneously aimed at the emotional level and the physical tissues. The premise of Russell and Stone that "thoughts are things" was reinforced again if one considered retained fears and thoughts. A common denominator in the work and ideas of all these thinkers and practitioners was their connection to respiration.

CHAPTER SIX

## Respiration Retraining

It has been said that the quality of one's respiration is rarely the cause for subjective reflection. It is often ignored, and the connection between subconscious repression of the breath and trauma can be missed. In his course notes, Fulford reflected:

> Strangely, many people actually turn against their breathing. Breathing itself has become an unnatural act for them, a stress, and a chore. Basic to all work on anyone's physical body, we must teach them to like breathing. And this is important because there is a constant balancing taking place between the vital regenerating force of the etheric matrix and the degenerative and decaying forces of the physical body and the environment.[20]

Fulford described a number of physical exercises that would enhance well-being. In particular, he liked to encourage the total enhanced respiratory response through a protocol he called the *piston breath*. The piston breath begins with an instruction to sit very erect, and to shift one's shoulders back as if in the military posture of "attention." Following this, the arms are brought back with the forearms in maximal supination. At this point of readiness, one begins a steady cadence of breathing without pause. Breath in, breath out, breath in, breath out . . . not rushing, but completely filling and emptying the lungs without pause. On the exhalation, one gets some progressive release of upper body tension and can take up the slack, or new flexibility, by engaging every aspect of the posture to a new barrier of resistance.[21]

The patient is told to practice this exercise once a day, trying to steadily increase the number of counts that could be endured. The maneuver was aimed at engaging, in a general way, any restriction to respiratory mobility, using the power of the lungs to promote freer motion.

It was Dingle, however, who directed Fulford's attention toward behavioral intervention to improve the breathing and its consequences on a physical, emotional, and spiritually developmental level. Dingle taught Fulford the value of respiratory self-training to increase one's vitality or youthfulness. Dingle, like Stone, had studied in Asia and there adopted the name Ding Le-Mei. In the 1950s, as part of an amalgam of eastern and western teachings, he taught the importance of pranic breathing at the Church of Mental Physics in Los Angeles. He and his followers operated the Institute of Mental Physics, a retreat in Yucca Valley near Palm Springs. The institute continues to distribute Dingle's material to this day. As previously noted, the Fulford family visited and participated in the program.

Dingle explained the importance of breathing in the context of a Hindu-based cosmology. He noted the importance in this system of a balance between the five vital airs or tattvas. Each had its complementary virtues and strengths, and together they supported the physical universe. Like Stone and Russell, rhythmic motion coincident with consciousness was part of the personal experience of being. This rhythm was linked to the breath cycle. Conscious breathing, by maximizing the energy exchange in the breath cycle, enhanced the integration of these principles.

Dingle also wrote in an aphoristic style. The following passages from his writings provide a sense of his message:

> The universe is simply one great, wonderful, vibrating, thinking thing.
>
> All Matter is electrical energy.
>
> You know that all energy, the energy that I use to think and write and the energy you use to think and read equally with the energy that you use in doing the work you perform, derives from one source…God, the Creator, the Divine Wisdom, the Creative Spirit, the Supreme Architect, the Primary Power, the indwelling, the Father.
>
> Every person will know that his body is an aggregation of cell life. It is gloriously more than that, for it is an aggregation of infinitesimally tiny universes of radiant energy, not matter as generally understood.[22]

These passages reflect the manner in which this evangelical thinker joined the materialistic and vitalistic principles into one potentially unified worldview. The functional application of this concept was the exercise of self-vitalization by more complete respiration. Dingle's view of the energetic universe and the energetic person was continuous with the eastern view of prana. Like food, respiration is nourishing. Prana is present everywhere as an ether; it is ingested through breath and nourishes us. The highest action of prana is thought. Thus, correct breathing enhances our consciousness, which is self-creative.

"Health involves correct thinking and correct breathing."[23] By "correct thinking," Dingle was referring to unified prayer or meditation. His system of correct breathing was represented by a sequence of exercises:

- revitalizing (complete) breath

- inspirational breath

- perfection breath

- vibro-magnetic breath

- cleansing breath

- grand rejuvenation breath

- your own spiritual breath

This system proved too complex for Fulford to use in his clinical work. Instead, he reformulated the principles into those of the piston breath (described above), and added intentionality to increase the effectiveness of the process.

### REFERENCES

1. Sutherland WG. *The Cranial Bowl.* Indianapolis, IN: The Cranial Academy, 1948 (orig. 1939): 24.

2. Ibid., 46.

3. Ibid., 56.

4. Ibid.

5. Magoun H. *Osteopathy in the Cranial Field,* 3rd ed. Indianapolis, IN: The Cranial Academy, 1976: 231.

6. Arbuckle BE. *The Selected Writings of Beryl E. Arbuckle.* Camp Hill, PA: National Osteopathic Institute and Cerebral Palsy Foundation, 1977.

7. Robert Fulford's course notebook (unpublished), page 15.

8. Ibid.

9. Robert Fulford's notebooks (unpublished).

10. Sutherland WG. *Teachings in the Science of Osteopathy*. Portland, OR: Rudra Press, 1990: 108-9.

11. Arbuckle, *Selected Writings*, 66-78.

12. Leboyer F. *Birth Without Violence*. New York: Alfred Knopf, 1975: 8.

13. Truby, The newborn baby's cry. *Acta Paediatrica Scandinavica* 1965 (supp.): 163.

14. Verny T. *The Secret Life of the Unborn Child*. New York: Dell Publishing, 1981: 20.

15. Ibid., 58-63.

16. Chamberlain D. *Babies Remember Birth*. Los Angeles: Jeremy Tarcher, Inc., 1988.

17. Diamond J. *Life Energy*. New York: Dodd Mead Company, 1985: 38.

18. Ibid.

19. Ibid., 48. The author here is referring to the Lung meridian of acupuncture.

20. Robert Fulford's personal notebooks (unpublished).

21. Ibid.

22. Dingle E. *Breathing Your Way to Youth*. Yucca Valley, CA: The Institute of Mental Physics, 1931.

23. Ibid.

PART THREE

# Fulford's Practice

"Your own native ability, with nature's book, are all that command respect in this field of labor. Here you lay aside the long words and use your mind in deep and silent earnestness; drink deep from the eternal fountain of reason, penetrate the forest of that law whose beauties are life and death. To know all of a bone in its entirety would close both ends of an eternity."

—*Andrew Taylor Still*

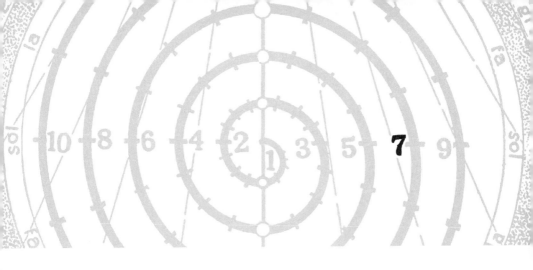

# 7

# Diagnosing with Dr. Fulford

## Introduction

*T*here are, of course, aspects of Fulford's work that are found in other approaches to osteopathic evaluation and treatment. However, the redefinition of the person, described in previous chapters, augmented Fulford's perception and was present in every aspect of his contact with his patients. The way in which he blended different emphases changed over the course of his career. As he became drained by the work of the treatments, as his intellectual development matured, and as his reputation attracted more difficult cases, Fulford chose to work in the ethric field much of the time. His unique methods themselves gradually attracted patients who had not responded to more conventional methods.

Practically speaking, how did Dr. Fulford implement this unique approach to the patient? Following the dictums of Dr. Still, Fulford came to view the physical body in tandem with a spiritual and mental body.[2] Since, as we have seen, Fulford viewed the physical body as the emanation or reflection of a higher level of organization, his method of screening was primarily aimed at discerning disturbances, and potential interventions, at multiple levels. Then he would discern the proper level of restriction, which he would deduce from his palpation of the physical body, ethric body, and emotional body.[3] Although he observed the movement of the abdominal diaphragm and the fascially disseminated effects of mechanical tension, his focus was elsewhere. Instead, he claimed to be palpating the electromagnetic aspect of the body directly. Sometimes he would do this while palpating the surface of the body, and sometimes by holding the hands off the skin surface.

Here we will discuss practical ways to catch up with Fulford. For us, following him means refocusing our attention during our basic palpatory contact with the patient.

*Demeanor and Style*

As we have seen, Dr. Fulford was an eclectic and intuitive physician who freely adapted the concepts and terminology of others. There was a fluidity with which he floated between paradigms in his evaluation. This occurred because his primary focus remained on the ethric body. In other words, Fulford felt that the results of trauma—reflected in residual dysfunction and pain—were primarily an assault on the ethric body; the physical symptoms were merely reflections of this assault. Perturbation of the field was often present even in a presymptomatic state. These perturbations could be detected because they restricted proper movement, and they could be released by standard osteopathic methods. However, when he used conventional technique, Fulford's methods of diagnosis and treatment followed the gentle articular techniques taught by Sutherland, which in turn were adapted from Still. They are described in Sutherland's *Teachings in the Science of Osteopathy.*[4]

In a patient, an unresolved residual dysfunction from prior failed treatments often represented a *blockage in energy flow.* This reflected both a subtle disturbance in the neuromuscular homeostasis and in the personal evolution of the person. Spiritual, psychological, or physical arrest in the individual's development could manifest in physical symptoms. The task of the diagnosing physician could be quite complex, especially with the difficult patient. And recall that it was the difficult patients who sought Dr. Fulford's help.

Fulford approached this challenge with each patient by following certain principles that we will try to illustrate, but he was also guided by his intuitive feeling for the person in front of him. In a sort of reverse transference, he would pay close attention to *his* feelings in response to the patient. Body language and voice tone, another expression of the life force of the patient, may reveal as much as the palpable findings.

Summing up his attitude toward assessment, Fulford once told a neighbor that his task in life was to become progressively more aware of the nature of his relationship to the patient. This was especially true of children, with whom he was empathetically bound and could establish rapport though the use of words, and infants, with whom he needed to relate on a preverbal level. Clearly, this was a multidimensional task. It was certainly not the cultural norm of medicine where visits to a physician are regarded as a product supplied by a "provider." I believe that the basis for this close physician-patient alliance was rooted in his own childhood conflicts, something to which he could still vividly relate.

In any case, each encounter included establishing rapport with the patient—his voice was strong and authoritative, but gentle and nurturing. He had a way of using colloquial language and joking with the patient to communicate his concern and his findings. In later years he took on a distinctly grandfatherly air, which made most people who were younger than himself (at 92, this would have included all his patients!) feel supported. His intention of giving loving service and working with the Creator provided an additional dimension to the encounters. Sometimes these elements took on a formulaic or ritualistic form, and sometimes they were tacit; however, they were always there.

*Spiritual Dimension*

Fulford was not theologically oriented in his approach to spirituality. He would not discuss the topic in a theological context. To me, this silence was significant. He would not discuss the issue beyond the need to recognize the presence and power of the Creator, especially in the areas of the being, health, and healing of the patient. When asked questions with religious implications, he would comfortably reply in general, humanistic terms. Moreover, the subject of religion was not broached in either course work or other educational settings. In a man whose thoughts were quite complex, and whose reading material was full of such discussions, there is an ambiguous message in this silence.

Some practitioners of subtle osteopathy intimate that all the action is in the spiritual or esoteric sphere. Fulford was able to address these same realities but bring them in line with the development of classical osteopathy. Still had created a foundation in osteopathy for integrating theological concepts. Sutherland was more subtle in the manner in which he incorporated the spiritual dimension, which he called the "potency," in his cranial work. Fulford also first raised this subject when he was learning the nuances of cranial osteopathy, and would often use the subtle articular, fascial, and respiratory relationships described by Sutherland. It is interesting that Fulford, like Sutherland, paid more attention to the empirical experience of engaging forces on all levels in the tissue than to discussions of theology.

*Evolving Ideas*

Fulford's diagnostic principles and methods underwent constant change, often weekly, even up to the final days of his life. As a result, some of his methods were highly variable. Throughout this book, I have highlighted two aspects of his evolving methodology. First, there is Fulford's emphasis while doing articular and connective tissue work, including in the cranial field, on consideration of the ethric field. Thus, even when Fulford applied what appeared to be classical osteopathic principles, including those of the interrelationship of structure and function, he had in mind working with the energetic activity of the patient, as reflected in the respiratory process and fascial mobility. Second, in his treatments, Fulford attempted to address the bioelectric properties of the field, which is not so obviously related to conventional osteopathy. In this he was influenced by such individuals as Stone and Johnston, discussed in Chapter 5, and others whom we will discuss in Chapters 9 and 10.

In the middle period of his life, when he was developing the theoretical explanation for the utility of the percussion vibrator, he hypothesized the presence of "energy sinks" to describe localized dysfunction. Thus, if healthy body tissue has an energetic wave characterized by harmonious flow, dysfunction dampens the wave, which represents a trauma-induced unresponsiveness to this harmonious process. By analogy, if you are soldering two pieces of metal with a torch and don't want the heat to pass further along the metal parts, you would use a clamp as a "heat sink" to absorb the heat. Identifying and treating these energy sinks is one way of describing Fulford's overall treatment objective.

### Who Is My Patient?

Fulford viewed the patient as an evolving composite of all their experiences, including their individual genetic expression, nutritional history, birth experience, and life events of all kinds, physical, emotional, and spiritual. The diagnostic process included attentive history-taking, observation, and palpation of the person for restriction of motion and tissue texture change, but also for turbulence in the ethric field. Fulford's judgment was largely based on intuition. The Doctor would work with his eyes closed, concentrating to perceive the body's message, and with a firm intention of simultaneously intervening, adjusting, and fine-tuning as he proceeded. The data he got was different from what we would use in most medical decision-making situations.

There is a tale of the man who came to him with a significant complaint. Fulford examined him briefly and sent him away saying he could not help in this case. Once the patient left, Fulford commented that he could not treat the man because he was already dead. Three days later, the man died. This was the exceptional case. I use it only to demonstrate that Dr. Fulford worked with calm assurance, using deep intuition from an inner forum. Having worked beside him on patients, I concluded that imitation was not the goal; rather, it was a question of cultivating one's own inner gifts. This brings us to the issue of the role of the physician.

### Physician as Facilitator

Much of Dr. Fulford's success came from his own cultivation as a facilitator for change in the patient. To engage the patient on the level required for the "work," the practitioner must cultivate him- or herself on a variety of levels. In addition, in the encounter with a patient, the practitioner might recognize that the treatment process is a reciprocal exchange on the physical, emotional, and energetic levels.

A significant amount of the preparation involves being aware. The physician's study sharpens the eye, mellows the heart, and makes his or her own field harmonious in preparation for engaging the patient.

### *Fulford's Personal Preparation*

Drawing on the analogy of tithing, a biblical reference to giving back to God one-tenth of one's gifts, Fulford took one-tenth of his day to "run the energy." That is, he would conceptualize the surface energy flow of the body described by Stone (see Figs. 4-3 through 4-5 in Chapter 4). He would awaken in the early hours of the morning, and for the next two-and-a-half hours would visualize and feel the flow of energy in his own body, first down the front and back up on the right, and then in the reverse direction on the left. Fulford typically retired early, because he awoke early. He recognized that when he treated difficult cases his own energy field was depleted. He used these and other exercises to increase his own breath, energy, and stamina to enable himself to be available and of use to others. At the same time, this exercise served as a form of meditation to strengthen his ability to concentrate and focus his intention, which was often the critical element in both diagnosis and treatment.

There is also the issue of the physician's energy field. The energetic polarity interaction that arises as a result of contact with the patient will be addressed below in our discussion of the physical examination. As we shall see, polarity exists even without contact. This interaction involves complementary contact, positive contacting negative.

## History-Taking

From our presentation thus far, the reader can see that Fulford's goals in diagnosis were to discover restrictions of motion, and, when it appeared appropriate, to discover a cause for those restrictions as well as what I call "restrictions of being."[5] Fulford dug deeply, trying to understand and incorporate into his treatments several issues raised by Still: the nature of "both ends of a bone," the Triune Man, and the question of "What is life?" The latter issue in particular is indeed a question to which Still paid considerable attention, but which we often decline to investigate. As previously noted, this question was the basis for Still's discussion of biogenic life, the union of the material and spiritual aspects of man.

Thus, Fulford had a head-full just from meeting a patient. Certainly he would want to know why the patient had come to see him, which is to say, a detailed history as described by the patient. He would listen to the history of prior diagnoses and treatment, and of remissions and exacerbations. The patient's expectations were also important. Then Fulford would look for other events: the history of trauma and birth experience led the list, especially since the two were related.

Trauma included falls and accidents, of course, but also personal violent contact. He probed beyond recent events, trying to discern the temporal association of the symptoms to stages of development in the patient. If the trauma affected the ethric body before the expression of physical symptoms, the lag between the associated events could be considerable. Fulford would begin by reviewing a detailed history of recent physical trauma and then proceed to review the individual's life in ten-year blocks. Often, later in the course of a treatment, a patient would remember a long-forgotten event, as if the softening of the flesh released memories long stored. Fulford knew that emotions and thoughts could galvanize the effects of stress. Such insights allowed the patient to accept and recognize the significance of the distant experience. This accentuated the effects of the treatment.

If the traumatic experience was identified, Fulford sought to determine whether there was any associated emotional content. What was on the person's mind at the time of the event, and what his or her emotional reaction to it? Was there resentment, fear, or anger toward the event or the perpetrator that was blocking the resolution of the physical expression of the symptoms? If the individual had no personal emotional reaction, were there strong emotions associated with the event in others that could have been transferred to the patient? Sometimes the nature of the trauma involved totally verbal or attitudinal contact; physical contact was not necessary.

An *in utero* traumatic event might be at the root of the patient's ills. Fulford also wanted to know about the physical experience of the birthing process, as this could leave an ethric and physical imprint on the individual. For most of us, birth represents a traumatic right of passage, and the stress of the birth is necessary to shock the infant into expressing its desire to thrive by way of the first independent breath. Even the position of the emerging infant's head might later direct the thoughts of the patient during the physical exam, especially in younger children.

In his work with developmentally disabled and delayed children, Fulford consistently tried to discern harmful prebirth experiences and accompanying emotional issues that could have originated from either parent to the child or between the parents. In addition, in cases involving children suffering from retardation, developmental delay, or malformation, Fulford often found that one or both parents transferred stressful or negative influences to the child through the ethric entity, which before and during the birthing process included both the mother and the fetus. In addition, an unexpected, inconvenient, or unwanted pregnancy—occasionally even a failed abortion—can have negative effects on infants. Financial or other difficulties can result in a restriction of form, function, or fullness of development. All of these factors represent the psychosomatic equivalent of the shared immunity that exists between the mother and fetus and between the mother and young child.

Fulford recognized that these factors represented part of the history, and sometimes the true cause, of his patients' symptomatology, and needed to be recognized before fuller healing could take place. All of this was done softly, but with a firm shifting of responsibility to the parents, or to the patient, about what to do next. In these cases, the osteopathic work was seen as secondary to the psychological and interpersonal work that was needed to rectify the ethric health of the individual. There was no sense of judgment or guilt imparted, just the urgency of the need to recognize the root of the problem and to correct it. Of course, osteopathic intervention could assist in this process by promising, when appropriately targeted, to help resolve associated dysfunctions and symptoms.

## Physical Examination

As if to leave a door open for all of us to use, Dr. Fulford would do a version of a musculoskeletal exam, compatible with many other systems, for analyzing the posture, gait, and structure of the patient. Doing a thorough conventional exam based on his training, he would initially pay attention to the region of the symptom. During this process, however, he would start to look for the appearance of patterns of dysfunction. Sometimes this would be guided by reflexes that he had been taught, which are no longer a part of the educational curriculum. An example would be the rhino-rectal reflex, which often appears to be relevant in an atopic person with chronic rhinitis and underlying sacral dysfunction. Fulford would also try to determine the constitution of the patient using methods that were based on the ideas of Brenda Johnston, Randolph Stone, Robert Becker, or Valerie Hunt. He would, for example, use Stone's reflections on "companion vertebrae" when he felt it was appropriate. Most of the time, however, he attributed patterns of dysfunction to the descent in the birth canal and to the delivery. Unless he found otherwise, he would assume that the patient was in the left-occiput-anterior position during the birthing process, and would evaluate the parts most particularly strained in this process (see Fig. 6-1 in Chapter 6).

In the birthing process, the head (occiput) takes much of the strain and emerges first. The shoulder comes next, followed by the left hip, with the left knee crossed over the right leg. Fulford would look for residual strain in these areas and for restriction in the movement of the left calcaneus, tibia, and patella.

During birthing, problems could occur that would affect the infant and later the adult. If there were restrictions in the fascia and membranes of the birth canal, it would not expand sufficiently. Another possibility is that the force of contractions would be lacking. In such cases there would be abnormal strain patterns put into the fascia and membranes of the child during the birthing process. These and other problems might ulti-mately compromise the capacity for movement and development in the infant and in the adult. In such cases, Fulford would find restrictions in subtle motions and in the ethric field. He would treat these restrictions using the breathing methods described in Chapter 6. These methods acted like the inflation of a balloon to help unfold the whole body and release the strains.

### Polarity

At times during the physical examination the use of hand polarity was emphasized. In Chapter 4 we alluded to the influence of Randolph Stone, but the issue is more complicated. His approach was influenced by the ideas of Stone as well as another individual, discussed below. Fulford emphasized the polarity of the examiner's hands, noting the changing complementary electromagnetic properties of patient and physician dur-ing their encounter.

During the seated and supine examination, Fulford followed the teachings of Randolph Stone regarding complementary polarity, that is, Fulford used his right hand to examine the patient's left side. When Fulford and the patient were face-to-face, this position would occur nat-urally. However, when he was behind the patient, his hands had to be crossed to maintain this arrangement. This was important to Fulford, especially in the context of a cranial examination. With very young chil-dren, this is easily accomplished by allowing the child to remain on the mother's lap, which is acceptable since they share a common field early in the child's life.

In Tucson, Fulford met a Mexican healer (whose name he did not record) who described a modification to the approach described above. He taught Fulford to reverse that approach when he worked with female patients since the energy moves around the umbilicus in a clockwise direction in males and in a counter-clockwise direction in females. This periumbilical relationship is associated with the birthing experience and the cutting of the cord, and it affects any stored trauma (in the form of pain) to the lumbar region.

Although Fulford taught this modified approach in his courses, he did not emphasize it in his practice. The exception was the supine examination of the thorax and ribs, which he almost always performed using the modification. In his courses as well, Fulford appeared to minimize the issue of gender-related reverse polarity several years after he started teaching the percussion vibrator course. He was also less concerned with the issue of hand placement during vibratory treatments.

*The Examination Sequence*

Fulford would first attend to his general impression of the form and posture of the patient:

> A physical body is, and has, its essential form in the body structures. A bio-energetic field exists around the body maintaining the balance and total functioning of the physical form. If we become attached to a thought process which has a high emotional content, the thought pattern will be locked into the bio-energetic field which surrounds the physical body. The physical body will manifest itself in a distorted pattern, i.e., a slumping of the shoulders, a shortening of a leg, a twisting of a body, a pulling of the muscles of an eye or mouth. If continued for an extended period of time, these patterns will become chronic and locked into the body form. Thoughts are things.[6]

After completing this general reflective inspection, he would proceed with a more detailed structural exam. He would look at the lumbosacral area from behind for sulcus depth and iliac crest heights.

"Okay, siddown," he would say in his resigned, calm, but softly gruff voice, a throwback to the era in which he grew up in "Cincinnata." He would check the range of motion of the shoulder while stabilizing the scapula and clavicle. This would be tested by gently cradling the flexed elbow and using it as a lever to passively extend the abducted shoulder while continuing the circular motion until the straightened elbow allowed the arm to come forward into horizontal position in front of the patient (Figs. 7-1 & 7-2). "Oh, you can't reach into the cookie jar so well, I see." In addition to glenohumeral mobility, he would be feeling for the quality and extent of free motion among the complex elements of the shoulder

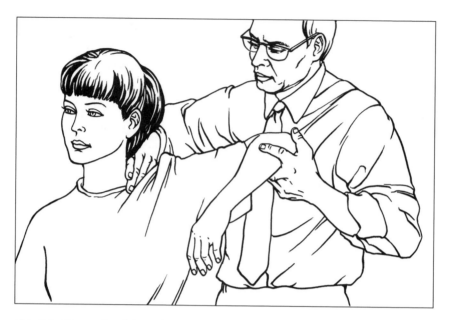

**Fig. 7-1** Diagnosis of thoracic outlet, the quality of respiration reflected in shoulder mobility—"getting into the cookie jar"

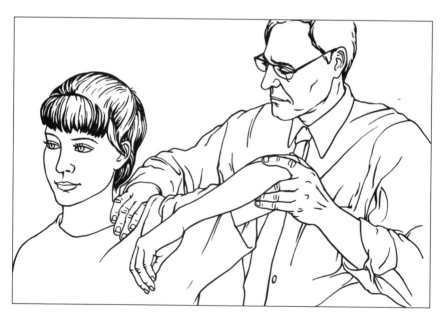

**Fig. 7-2** Diagnosis of respiration at thoracic outlet reflected in shoulder mobility—"getting into the cookie jar"

joint and their relation to the chest in full respiratory excursion. He was guided in part by the direction of energy flow described in Stone's *Wireless Anatomy of Man*, but he was also interested in what he called the "east-west axis," the laterally extended (abducted to horizontal) upper extremities.

*Supine Examination*

Next would come "Okay, lie down on the table." With the patient lying supine, Fulford would start at the feet, cradling each of the slightly raised heels in the palms of his hands. He would apply a gentle rhythmic rocking to determine the side of restriction, drawing inferences about hip function and pelvic mechanics from the end of the extremity resting in his hand (Fig. 7-3). He would emphasize that he was attending to subtle sensations of easing and binding, not to gross range of motion, sensing the restrictions in the tissues while accepting them simultaneously as an assessment of fluidity in the field.

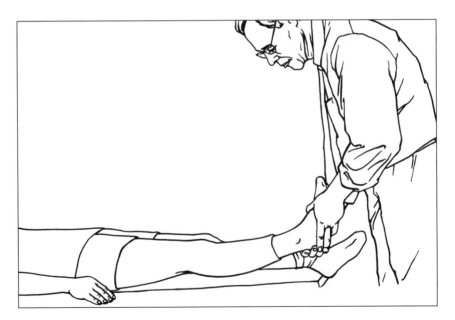

**Fig. 7-3** Diagnosis of lower limb, regional

Changes to the left knee in particular were included in the initial stage of Fulford's assessment, since any dysfunction of the knee might represent a residual effect of the birth trauma. He would check the knees by looking for a shift in the placement of the patella while the extremity rested on the table (Fig. 7-4). He would test each knee with a subtle lateral

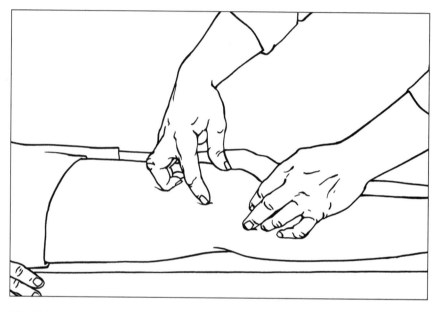

**Fig. 7-4** Diagnosis of patellar tracking

motion while lightly grasping the patella between the thumb and index finger. Then he would rock the pelvic bones by placing gentle pressure over the anterior superior spines (Figs. 7-5 & 7-6). He viewed this as a regional evaluation and made inferences about sacral mechanics from this position. Restriction to rocking meant articular restriction as well as restriction to energy flow. He would assess the sacrum in the lateral recumbent position, ignoring its position and attending instead to tissue resistance, which reflected field turbulence.

The abdominal area was assessed to determine the direction of the periumbilical flow of energy, especially the left subcostal area. Here, since it is unsupported by the liver, the abdominal wall may potentially reflect

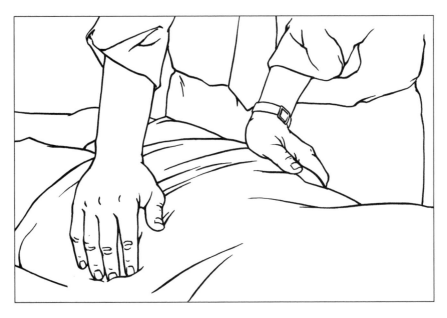

**Fig. 7-5** Diagnosis of pelvis with correct polarity

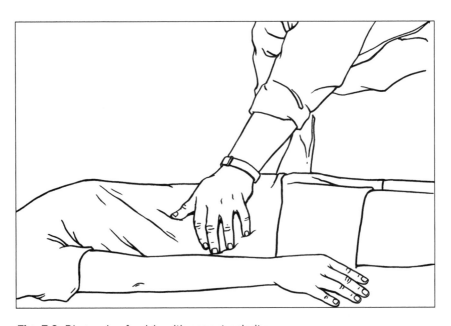

**Fig. 7-6** Diagnosis of pelvis with correct polarity

tension in the diaphragm, which Fulford termed the "shock of trauma." We will revisit this later, because it was often a focus of treatment for Fulford.

When the shock of trauma occurs in any part of the body the rhythm of the breath becomes disturbed. The diaphragm is restricted and locked up under the body of the sternum. The shock will produce a small recess the size of one's little fingernail. It will only be found on the left side of the body of the sternum at the level of the sixth rib, or on a level with the xyphoid process where it attaches at the sternal body. This is very diagnostic for locating a shock in the body, even when the patient doesn't remember the incident.

Fulford would also assess the expansion of the rib cage by conforming his fingers to the shape of the ribs and placing them lightly on the rib cage as the patient breathed naturally. He would look for a "dip" or depression on the right lateral chest wall, between ribs 5 and 7, indicative of a shock being locked in the body (Fig. 7-7). Alternatively, the shock, which rep-

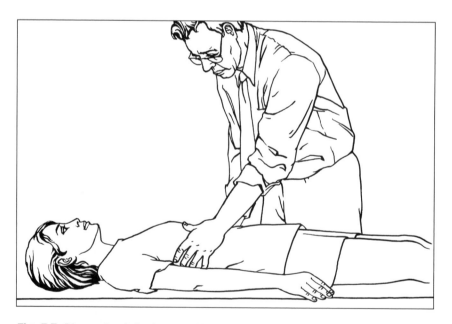

**Fig. 7-7** Diagnosis of diaphragm with correct polarity, resulting from shock or trauma

resents a restriction in the field affecting the respiratory process, may manifest as a small recess on the right arm (Fig. 7-8). Why the right side? Fulford gave no reason other than this was his experience—sometimes that was just the way he worked.

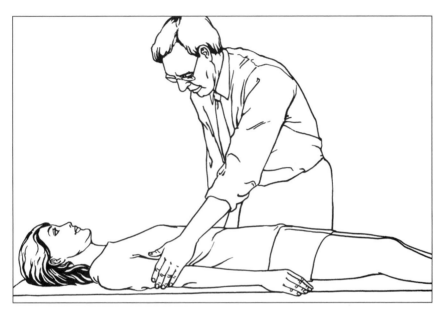

**Fig. 7-8** Diagnosis of lateral arm with correct polarity, resulting from shock

Standing in front of the patient, Fulford would assess the cervical spine by using gentle articular motion, drawing inferences about the state of the Breath. As he probed higher and higher, eventually reaching the tissues above the shoulders, his focus centered more and more on the breath. His reinterpretation of the significance of respiration changed his thinking about the goals of cranial palpation and manipulation (Fig. 7-9). Early in his training and career, he felt that the key lay in unfolding the membrane and cartilages of the head. However, as previously noted, Fulford was aware that Sutherland was questioning the nature of the force behind the continuously flowing cerebral spinal tide, which he compared to "Liquid Light."[7] Fulford was also acquainted with Walter Russell's

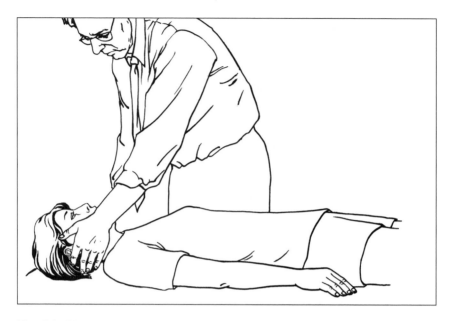

**Fig. 7-9** Diagnosis of cranium and cervical spine with correct polarity

notion that the "highest known element" included a creative power, which in many respects was analogous to light. Another important concept of Russell's was that the creative intent was carried out by word, intention, and will, which he felt were the bases for love. By joining these ideas to the Hindu concept of the nutritional power of respiration—prana— Fulford came to see an association among a person's strength to fulfill his or her potential (beginning at birth), vitality (as expressed in his or her respiration), and the level of resonance in their electromagnetic field.

So while his colleagues were palpating the cranium looking for the expression of the Cranial Rhythmic Impulse, Fulford, at a later stage in his development, was looking for other kinds of information. His cranial exam focused on certain key elements beyond the mobility and relationship of the sphenobasilar junction, the coiling of the brain, the membranous tension, and the fluctuation of the fluids. His interest in the global issues of vitality and mobility, as well as respiration and the manner in which it expressed itself as a person developed, led him to emphasize:

• mobility of the zygoma and the nasal reflection of the ethmoid

- mobility of the occiput and its relationship to the mobile sacrum

- energy or breath flowing to the top of the vault, or through that region via the falx to the anterior portion of the cranium and face.

Because of the oscillatory and circular nature of this energy flow—from the anterior cervical fascia and sternum in the sagittal plane to the clavicles, shoulders, and upper extremities in the coronal plane—Fulford would pay special attention to any palpable dysfunction in these areas.[8]

Based on his understanding of embryology (discussed below), Fulford attached considerable importance to the area of the anterior chest and face, from the sternum to the mouth and nose and from the frontal bone to the occiput. According to Fulford, this area reflects events that individuals experience while they are still in the embryonic stage. However, this is at variance with orthodox cranial practice, which tries to determine the potential mobility (or restriction) of the deeper dural aspects of the cranium as well as the fluid and articular relationships of the vault. Fulford went beyond Sutherland's concept of potency, palpating this area to determine the potency of the Life Force as expressed in the L-field (see Chapter 3). For Fulford, this was a practical clinical application of those principles. The implications seemed to be of particular importance to Dr. Fulford, partly on behalf of his patients, but also partly because of the pressure he felt for holding this unorthodox view.

## Which End Is Up?

*Interpreting the Impact of Fetal Development on the Individual*

The subtle relationships of the body reflect the ethric, emotional, and spiritual components in the adult as well as in the individual's early development, starting from the moment of conception. Some embryologists recognize an electromagnetic axis with a positive charge at the cranial pole as an organizing force in the early embryologic stage of tissue differentiation and migration.[9]

The location of the sternum over the heart center has its embryological origins in the anterior pole of the embryonic plate, and perhaps in part

105

of the yolk sac as well, even before the differentiation of the nervous system. The precordial enfolding brings this electromagnetic pole portion of the embryo into its adult location on the anterior part of the trunk, integrating the heart center, or chakra, and the heart as an organ. This pattern has physical and energetic consequences, and is consistent with Becker's measurements in salamanders and humans. As a result, Fulford would, in certain patients, scrupulously look for perturbations in the field and altered respiratory patterns on the anterior aspect of the body.

Certainly, the mouth and nose are intimately involved with the first breath. The nasal passage and nasal bones not only admit air but are also in direct contact with the brain through the olfactory bulb. Traditional cranial osteopathy considers this to be an area of importance because of the anterior insertion of the falx cerebri at the crista galli, allowing for mobility of the ethmoid, vomer, and nasal bones. Fulford, however, recognized a continuum of influences down to the precordial level. His multilevel interest in the anterior thoracic area, for example, is reflected in a letter written the year before his death:

> Thanks for your letter, I am glad that I could help you. That is what fifty-four years of practice has produced.
>
> Osteopathy has a philosophy of 'We are a Spiritual being, a Mental being and have a material body.' Cause is in the Spiritual and Mental and the effect is in the material. Most doctors treat the effect.
>
> The thymus gland monitors and regulates energy flow throughout the body. Wherever an imbalance occurs, it rebalances the energy. The thymus is the first organ of the body to be affected by stress, whether it is physical stress—infection, disease—or mental stress. It is the link between the mind and the body.[10]

Here he is relating the deeper significance of the cranium to the idea of the energy centers in general, and the importance of the heart center in particular. While his thoughts on the sternum were based in part on the teachings of Brenda Johnston and others, Fulford developed his own protocol by blending Sutherland's method of subtly reading the body with Vogel's manner of manipulating energy, a subject discussed in Chapter 9. It is nevertheless important to point out here that Vogel considered the thymus to be significant in the emotional organization of the body, and that Vogel's clinical approach involved the use of a crystal; Fulford used his hands to the same end. Thus, for Fulford, the sternal precordial area was a point of primary interest in his diagnosis and treatment methods.

To evaluate this area, Fulford would stand in front of the patient, who was seated or supine, and place his left hand to the right side of the head and his right hand to the left side of the head. He would then evaluate the nasal area, the zygomata bilaterally, and the sphenoid, temporal, frontal parietals and occiput, looking for restrictions in mobility as well as blockages to the flow of energy. He was adamant about this approach, and he persevered in promoting it before The Cranial Academy even in his last address to that body (see Appendix B).

As previously noted, Fulford saw a relationship between the shoulder and the cranial areas from a structural, functional, and energetic point of view. Recall that in his cranial palpation, Fulford would be looking for articular restrictions, but more importantly, he wanted to find a full, deep "breath," a feeling of expansiveness that reached from the crown to the front portion of the head. This would indicate that the ethric body, the L-field, was fully energized with vital force.

### How Does One Palpate the Ethric Field?
### What Does It Feel Like?

In his "energy work," Fulford maintained that the two hands work together, even while using the percussion vibrator. This differs from the convention of having a motor hand and a monitoring hand, which is common in some other aspects of osteopathic work. Additionally, he joined his mental faculties—his intention—to complete the therapeutic triangle (two hands plus intention). He referred to making the triangles discussed in the works of Brenda Johnston and Randolph Stone. Fulford advised us to do this as well, but without offering an explanation. Let me offer my interpretation of what Fulford meant, in the form of two exercises, since it is easier to demonstrate through empirical exercises than it is to explain.

## Palpating Field Contours *(per Z. Comeaux)*

Sit comfortably and quietly, by yourself. Relax and allow your mind to become calm. Watch your breathing or "center" in whatever fashion you find natural. A peaceful atmosphere in which to do this work is helpful.

If you are experienced in any type of meditation then you are aware of an inner "place" of peace that you can visit at will. With practice, you can visit this "inner forum" no matter how chaotic the environment is outside you. In meditation, one sometimes uses a mantra, a repeated word or phrase, to help in the centering process, distracting oneself from the routine cognitive processes. I have used visual mantras, such as a pleasant picture in the treatment room, as a visual equivalent. Eventually, you will want to center yourself without external aids.

From this quiet place, let your arms hang at your side. Then bend your elbows, allowing your open palms to face one another but remain separated at approximately shoulders' width. Now, slowly allow them to approach one another and explore what you feel in the space between. Especially if you have done palpatory work, at some point you will sense a certain interface, a change in texture, a subtle barrier.

If you were to put your hands into very cold water, it would be easy to sense the entry point with your eyes closed. As you lower the temperature differential between the body and the water to a degree or two, the nature of the task changes. A more subtle transition requires more concentration and perhaps some practice. The experience of these field contours is an exercise of this nature. Trust your intuition and just accept what you feel, without analysis or judgment. Practice pays off.

Next, place one palm facing the front of your chest with the arm extended. Move slowly toward the chest and note what you feel. Note any qualitative change, then repeat to verify or modify your perception. Do this same exercise with a confidant who will not report you for being crazy. If you are currently in practice, make a habit of checking the field contours with your hand behind the patient's back until you feel comfortable talking about what you are doing.

If possible, do this exercise on patients who are obviously debilitated, such as those with a serious illness, significantly upset, demented, or schizophrenic. In my early learning, I would palpate fields during nursing home rounds on people who were struggling with serious chronic conditions. Over time, you begin to get a sense of interpersonal differences, similar to your experiences when you were new to osteopathic training and palpating. Once you develop this facility you can use it to make region-to-region comparisons within the person and to note changes during treatment.

## Triangulation: Joining the Hands and Heart

Center in whatever way is comfortable for you. Breathe in and out peacefully. Put your attention into your breathing. Sit with your hands supported on your lap, resting. Now shift your attention to your left hand, paying attention to what it feels like. Create an "eye," a center of attention in your left palm. Now do the same in the right palm and have the two "look" at one another. In other words, be aware of the sensations of each hand simultaneously and have them feel each other at a distance.

Now, pay attention to the place of emotion in your chest, behind your sternum. If you have trouble with this, think of a very nice or a very bad thing that has happened to you and see where you feel it originate. Pay attention to this place and to your hands at the same time. These three points of awareness—the sternum (heart center) and two palms—create a powerful instrument from which to note changes in patients. They act as a committee of surveillance. You can shift your attention from one point of the triad to another during palpation and get a deeper sense of what you feel and the degree of concurrence or disagreement. This is a powerful tool for beginning to sense the patient on a deeper level.

Once you become familiar with this method of palpating, you may occasionally find that the quality of input from one hand or from your heart may not be at its best some of the time. You may find that you have a "dominant hand"—which may not be identical to your handwriting handedness—whose perceptions sometimes seem clearer. The sensitivity may be adjusted by your intentional focus, a form of concentration. If not, it is good to recognize when one is limited in one's effectiveness and choose another means of assessing patients.

In any case, this awareness creates an attention center of its own that can be linked again through intention with the center of experience of the patient and with the "Higher Power" to create a still more powerful triad for diagnosing and treating. Recall Sutherland's admonition to develop seeing, feeling, knowing, and thinking fingers, a recognition of the enhanced synesthesia in palpation. Also his advice to stay close to your maker suggests the need to include the Higher Power in the diagnostic and treatment processes.

Intention and awareness are important for a number of reasons. From his study with Russell and Stone, Fulford firmly believed that thoughts are things. Thoughts and words can inflict trauma, but they are also currency for one's relationship with the patient that can be used to recruit the individual to his or her own healing. Thoughts are also the diagnostic and treatment tools that powerfully extend our efforts into the work needed for evaluating and working with the ethric field. Empathic recognition of buried conflict can be a liberating and health-inducing experience for the patient.

Thus, diagnosis is insight, not only in the sense of logical analysis or problem solving. Fulford maintained throughout that thoughts had therapeutic impact that began with thoughtful appreciation and attention to the patient at every available level. Hence his insistence on focused attention and purity of intention.

The diagnostic sequence described above adapts the subtle artic-ular way of working to the methods used in working with field dynamics. At times Fulford would focus almost entirely on field dynamics. He could do this with hand contact that was similar to one used for light palpation, or he could do it slightly off the body, contacting only the ethric field. I cannot describe to you what he felt; there was a limit to the Doctor's expressive talent. Refer to the palpatory exercises described here and you will head in the right direction. The preferred way to learn this art is by first practicing hand contact with a mentor, and with feedback.

## REFERENCES

1. Still AT. *Autobiography of A.T. Still.* Indianapolis, IN: American Academy of Osteopathy, 1981 (orig. 1908): 152.

2. Still AT. *The Philosophy and Mechanical Principles of Osteopathy.* Kirksville, MO: Osteopathic Enterprise, 1992 (orig. 1902): 16.

3. The terms ethric field, energy, L-field, Life Breath, or just "The Breath" are used interchangeably here. The term "emotional body" was coined by Brenda Johnston (see Chapter 4).

4. Sutherland WG. *Teachings in the Science of Osteopathy.* Portland, OR: Rudra Press, 1990.

5. This term, which I coined, refers to an arrest in the personal development of the patient, preventing the attainment of his or her potential.

6. Robert Fulford's basic and advanced percussion course notebooks (unpublished), page 22. These courses were presented at many venues, by invitation, between 1986 and 1997.

7. Sutherland WG. *Contributions of Thought.* Sutherland A, Wales A (small eds.) Fort Worth, TX: Sutherland Cranial Teaching Foundation, 1967: 347.

8. This is not the place to explore basic cranial osteopathy. Two good sources for this subject are Magoun HI. *Osteopathy in the Cranial Field,* 3rd ed. Indianapolis, IN: The Cranial Academy, 1976; and Chaitow L. *Cranial Manipulation Theory and Practice.* Kent, United Kingdom: Churchill-Livingston, 1999.

9. Nuccitelli R. "Endogenous Electric Fields in Developing Embryos." In *Electro-magnetic Fields*. Blank M (ed.) Washington, D.C.: American Chemical Society, 1995: 109.

10. Robert Fulford, unpublished letter to patient, 1997.

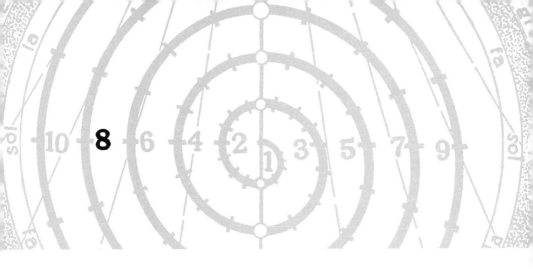

# 8

## Treating in the Style of Dr. Fulford

### Describing Fulford's Methods

*I* should like to begin this chapter by making it clear that Fulford practiced and taught as an American osteopathic physician. That is, he had been trained in medicine and surgery in addition to osteopathic manipulation; he himself would not train anyone who was not a physician. I present this material to share Fulford's experience and point of view, writing primarily for physicians. The techniques described below presume a background in osteopathic training.

One corollary to this is that, should you try to integrate any of these techniques or strategies into your own field of work, it is understood that basic medical diagnosis and treatment are part of the plan. To use these techniques outside that context is inappropriate and can put a patient at risk of serious harm. They do not represent an independent treatment system. Although Fulford diagnosed and treated in a somewhat unique way, he sought conventional medical diagnosis and treatment at appropriate times for himself, his family, and his patients.

Even in his courses, Fulford did not say a lot about the experience of treating. He would give general principles, particular guiding models, and affirmations and corrections regarding hand positions. But there were long silences, suggestions, and gaps in the details. In this chapter I will try to fill in some of these gaps to make it easier for the beginning student. I was myself a student and colleague of Dr. Fulford's for several years, which included frequent discussions, observing treatments, being a patient myself, treating the Doctor and his wife, as well as participating in workshops. I also participated in discussions for preparation of the book *Dr. Fulford's Touch of Life*. And again, after Fulford's death, I was privileged to receive and review the stacks of personal papers, correspondence, and source materials left by the Doctor. Yet I am reluctant to add too much by way of interpretation and surmise.

For example, I have tried to translate the experience of the energy field into particular experiential terms. Fulford never did this. Even when treating with him, I would be asked "Did you feel that?" but he would offer nothing more by way of description. Often Fulford would simply tell you to follow the energy.

There was a lot of subjectivity about his approach, which makes it difficult for me to elaborate without inventing. My descriptions here are drawn from being told by Fulford that I was "getting it," from positive feedback when I treated him or from the way I would describe what I felt and did, as I am doing here. But when a comment relies on significant interpretation of my own, it will be identified as such.

## Osteopathic Technique

From Dr. Still's time onward, osteopathic physicians have striven to base the techniques they use on the condition of the patient being treated. Rules that are based on anatomy and physiology, or the practice of other physicians, are helpful and necessary, but never sufficient. Recall that Fulford's overall goal was to discover blockages and release them. As noted earlier, the diagnosis might focus on restrictions in the articular aspect or directly on the ethric field. In this way, the healer would practically apply the osteopathic concept of triune nature to the patient, treating the physical body, the spiritual body, and the mind as one entity.

The physical body is engaged through hand contact with the appropriate fascial and articular parts of the body. The spiritual body is engaged by a centering and invocation, as described in Chapter 7.

At least during the time of his life when I knew him, Fulford was very centered. He had few interests outside the scope of the work described here. His general disposition was one of trust in the Creator, goodwill to all, a desire to serve and to heal. He did not pray in a formal sense, although he felt his life to be a gift from the Creator, and his daily meditation or preparation involved a commitment to tithe a tenth of his day to "running the energy," described in Chapter 7. From the time he arose, Fulford would maintain this energy consciousness throughout the day. When he treated, he would simply close his eyes to concentrate more clearly on the energy dimension, where he would feel for subtle flow or turbulence.

When working with crystals, after the pattern of Marcel Vogel, an actual invocation to the Creator to "charge the crystal" was a formal part of the preparation. Another part of Fulford's centering involved his disposition toward the patient. Through the history, he would concentrate on the experience of the patient by empathetically identifying with them. This was especially true of children. His whole affect and the tone of his voice would soften, and he would often seem to be in a reverie with the young patient.

I would like to begin with some observations about Fulford's method of working. The healer's mind is engaged by his intention to have a certain facilitative effect. Fulford described the need to "work in one's intention," both in the sense of generally wishing the patient well and of intervening on a specific level in the physical and ethric bodies.[1] This requires the development and conservation of one's own strength. Since the key level of engagement is with the field through intention, hand contact will vary from off-the-body palpation to light touch to conventional surface contact. Having stood by Fulford's side during many treatments, I can tell you that my best efforts working in his shadow came from performing the exercises described at the end of Chapter 7. These are derived from the concepts presented by Fulford in his 1988 introductory course, coupled with elements from the course in esoteric healing presented by Barbara Briner, D.O., who, like Fulford, experienced the teaching of Brenda Johnston.

When I worked with Fulford, beginning with conscious centering, I would concentrate on joining my own two hands to my heart center, and these to the seat of consciousness; I would then engage the patient as a similarly organized whole. For the invocation, I would intentionally join our two balanced selves to the Higher Power through our crown centers. I would then ask for help—beneficent assistance for goals beyond my comprehension. Then we—the physician together with a higher power—went to work, in cooperation with the patient.

I have expressed this in the language of my own experience. It reflects the composite influence of a number of the Doctor's teachers. Fulford always spoke as if the facts and findings were obvious; rarely did he make more than minimal reference to basic principles. Of course, to the learners who were working with him it was *not* always obvious, and Fulford would remark that the difference between them was fifty years of practice. I have always found it helpful to put my subjective reflections into words, but Fulford rarely did this. Hopefully, I have remained faithful to his intentions.

## Treatment Strategies

Based on my observation, Fulford had three treatment strategies:

1. He might address the immediate problem directly; this was only occasionally done, and then usually "on the road." Fulford would use a gentle articular technique, a direct connective tissue mobilization technique, an adjunct modality, such as percussion or magnets, or inductive intention to influence the patient's field locally. (The term *inductive intention* is defined under item three below.)

2. Fulford might begin with the focal complaint, but look for regional associations tied to the history and energetic constitution of the person. This approach was used more often than the first. Fulford was also oriented to the tradition of general treatment, which was then tailored to the individual patient. Since Fulford viewed somatic dysfunction as resulting from a blockage in energy flow, the treatment centered on removing the

blockage and facilitating the restoration of flow. Fulford's approach paralleled Still's, but with a twist: Still focused on restoring unimpeded arterial flow or unimpeded nerve force, while Fulford focused on restoring unimpeded flow in the ethric body. Both of them reviewed the "anatomy" and rectified suboptimal relationships to restore normal function. Fulford also followed the tradition of tailoring a general treatment to the specific needs of the individual patient.

3. The final treatment strategy can best be described by the use of a term I coined: *inductive intention.* Fulford often told us to heal by intention, but he only spoke in fragments about the nuts and bolts of this method. Having reviewed his sources, particularly Sutherland, Russell, Stone, and Vogel, I arrived at the term inductive intention and a description of how to do it. Following this strategy, Fulford would describe moving energy around to overcome blockages. These tasks are metaconceptual, or beyond complete description, but the work is real. If you sincerely toy with the words and concepts described here, you should meet the Force that is really doing the work—when you are invited. The concept of Force comes from the line of thought of Still, Sutherland, and Russell, all of whom viewed the patient's existence and state of well-being as the work of a personal Creator or personal God. Thus, the capacity to work on this level is partly a matter of talent, partly a matter of practice, and partly a matter of submitting oneself to serve the patient and to cooperate with the process that is actually in charge—when and if you are invited. This is not to say that there is a status attached to being accepted. Fulford himself recognized that the required skill is partly gift, partly a calling, and always the result of disciplined practice. He felt the work to be both a blessing to participate in and a burden. He said that contact with patients sapped his energy. He spoke of the rejection of his point of view by others within and outside of the profession. But he practiced with a grin of satisfaction.

The task of working with intention retraces the steps described in Chapter 7 on palpating the field. We need to center ourselves, to sense ourselves and our patients, to unite our centers with theirs, and to be open to help from the Creator. Once contact is made, we perform the diagnosis, looking for restrictions, just as all osteopaths are trained to do. Except, in this work, we are searching for the stirring and movement of the biodynamic field, the L-field, and trying to work with it. Any motion testing is subtle motion testing. Try to understand this approach by comparing it to the use of direct and indirect techniques. We can try to treat the physical restrictions using direct techniques. Alternatively, we can follow the dynamic motion to a position of balance, hold on to it, and monitor it until a spontaneous release occurs. Regardless, our goal should be to attain a sense of increased vitality, potency, or respiratory fullness. However, this is palpated in the gauzy texture of the field—with or without skin contact—not in the firm texture of the fascia, membranes, or musculoskeletal elements of the physical body. "Can one feel that?" you ask. By analogy, an amateur guitar player will tune the guitar near to correct pitch, but there may still be a slight dissonance, or pattern of discord, between supposedly identical notes on adjacent strings. A more skilled musician will be able to hear this, and recognize the need for further fine-tuning. Palpation of the field is something like that: you need to acquire an ear, and that takes practice, lots of practice.

## Treatment Methods

Fulford worked by engaging the patient on three levels and applying what I interpret to be three levels of "force" in his treatments: physical, energetic, and intentional. Each level of force, however, is simply a means of facilitating change, as if Fulford were dancing with the patient, rather than inducing a "correction." Regardless of which level of treatment was used, determining the end point relied on constant palpatory feedback.

1. The first level involved gentle guidance of tensions in connective tissue, including articular ligaments. Fulford would treat to balance these forces. This is most easily seen as an implementation of his training in cranial osteopathy and related fields. He relied on a keen awareness of the

relevant anatomy, including that of the cranium. However, he translated his active motion testing into the level of subtle motion testing; his passive motion testing blended with palpation of the ethric body, described next.

2. The second level of engagement was at the electric or ethric level (see discussion of palpating the field in Chapter 7). When working at this level, you can feel resonance or disharmony in everything you touch, as you encounter other textures and resistance. I have noticed that as you make a conscious effort to become centered, you create a harmonious resonance in your own field. By recalibrating your sense of touch to cultivate this extra sense, your world is opened up to another realm of objective but only subtly palpable reality. Then, as you make hand contact with the patient, you can use your own field to facilitate a resonance or harmonious flow in the patient's field. Most often this is done while using a manual technique, one that is recognizable as physical work. However, since the attention of the practitioner is in the ethric body, the release is felt as a change of state. For example, Fulford would often be thrown off the body as a result of what he would call a "flip" in the tissues. I have not experienced that kind of release myself. However, when working together with Fulford, I have experienced a change in tension or in the respiratory rhythm, or a general feeling of well-being or *calming of turbulence,* at the same time that Fulford was thrown off, signaling the end of the treatment.

3. The third level is the use of intention. This partly involves an earnest attention to the details of what is happening to the patient, which includes visualizing the problem and the potential solution. In addition, Fulford always maintained the desire to benefit the patient and to pay attention to that task, as well as a desire to ask for help. This was sensed either in the heart aspect of the palpating triad or at a higher center.

I will add that Dr. Fulford had a consistent but reserved way of describing this process; many of the descriptive words and phrases used here are my own, having worked beside him, read his source materials, and discussed the concepts with him at length. In our frequent conversations, I would grope, as others have, to realize what Fulford's terse descriptions meant. Most often he would respond with little more than "that's right"; he was more a man of action than of words.

Underlying the clinical problem and treatment solution, there is the issue of the spiritual evolution of the patient. Life is a mystery beyond our comprehension. Especially in difficult cases, successful osteopathic work involves a willingness to cooperate in the ongoing creation of the individual. Recognition of the role of the Creator, or Life Force, is an essential part of the treatment. How one progresses in this quest is beyond the scope of this book.

## A Sample of Fulford's Approach to Treatment

Since Fulford's actual treatments varied a great deal, it may be useful to describe a typical general treatment. This approach was used routinely in his course presentations since it gave the beginner a tangible and orderly way in which to approach common problems. If you are familiar with the tradition of general treatment, you know that it will vary to meet the needs of the individual patient.

Fulford's methods tended toward assessing the patient using regional association of major joints or articulations. The maneuvers involved range-of-motion exercises that focus our attention on the energetic nature of the restrictions. In the end, articular release was achieved by disengaging the restriction on several planes simultaneously, as described in the previous section. The actual exercises are derived from Sutherland's approach, described in *Teachings in the Science of Osteopathy*,[2] which in turn relied on Still's technique, as revived by Van Buskirk.[3] Note, however, that the approach here focuses on discovering and dissolving the concentric energetic levels of the dysfunction. Because we are providing a general treatment, a protocol is followed, but with the recognition that our attention and effort will shift depending on what is discovered when we engage the person and his or her body. What follows, therefore, parallels the diagnostic sequence developed in the last chapter. The two can be intertwined in actual application.

*Treatment Sequence and Emphasis*

Begin the treatment with the patient in a supine position, starting with the feet, the energetic connection of the body to the earth. As described in our discussion of Randolph Stone's ideas (Chapter 4), the body consists of circulating loops of energy that travel from the head to the toes; the lower portion of the body represents a negative pole, balanced by the positive pole of the upper body, with the pelvis as a neutral balance point. Treatment of imbalances depends on opening these circuits to contact with the larger world, with grounding. Fulford would therefore start with the lower extremity, standing at the foot of the table, and cradle the patient's heel, thereby suspending the leg and thigh. He would assess by doing subtle motion testing, judging the very earliest response to motion, a sort of suspended jiggle.

As noted in Chapter 7, Fulford looked for a regional restriction pattern involving the ankle, knee, and hip. If he found one, he would direct his intention and attention toward releasing the restriction, while gently rocking the cradled heel in an oscillatory fashion. The rhythmic motion may induce progressive ligamentous loosening, resonating simultaneously on the physical and energetic planes. To restore midline tracking of the patella and balance the hip articulation at the same time, Fulford would hold the knee and confine the patella with one hand. He would flex the knee and hip and then extend the limb along three successive pathways: external rotation of the hip, internal rotation of the hip, and a neutral position. Each pass would terminate with a slight, gravity-induced snap of the supported knee. He would then recheck to verify that blockage to energy flow was removed.

He would then treat the pelvis and sacrum as a regional unit from the front, making hand contact on the anterior superior iliac spines. He would use this contact to gently rock the regional unit, with the intention of releasing energy. Unless he reverted to a more mechanical approach to the pelvis in response to a focal trauma, this served as his treatment of this part of the body. He would also frequently use the percussion vibrator on the right trochanter, as described in Chapter 9. In young children he would use the percussor to "give them a good spanking," applying the device to the sacrum with the intention of gently but firmly inducing a greater, freer respiratory excursion in the whole body.

According to Fulford, the abdominal area is a complex affair. As noted in Chapter 7, the periumbilical area is associated with the connection and separation issues that arise at birth. It could also be connected to back pain. If he thought this was germane in a particular patient, Fulford would lightly follow the flow of energy in the periumbilical area, trying to sense the degree of freedom and restriction; he would then use inductive intention with light contact to normalize the flow.

Because of its fascial connections, the subcostal or epigastric area reflects the respiratory activity of the thoracoabdominal diaphragm. Fulford also regarded the solar plexus as a visceral brain: a seat of emotion and a major energy center. Changes in this area are discernible in both its field contours and fascial tension, and its surface was a significant site for diagnosis and work in cases involving emotional trauma. Fulford was concerned about the shock that arose from trauma, especially in light of Pert's findings regarding the importance of neuropeptides (see Chapter 3). Fulford believed that a vast body of evidence substantiated the ancient wisdom of attending to the energy centers, the charkas. "Taking out the shock" associated with this area (described in Chapter 7) was an important element in a great number of Fulford's difficult cases, those which had resisted prior attempts at treatment. Again, it should be pointed out that, although the treatment described below superficially represents a myofascial procedure, it has other significant ramifications.

Fulford would stand on the left side of the patient with his fingertips aligned just left of and lateral to the linea alba. Following the breath (the actual exhalation of the lungs), Fulford would allow his hands to sink into the tissue of the abdomen and to hold the tension created through successive breath cycles until he felt a strong responsive respiratory effort reflecting enhanced vitality in the life field. He would usually do this treatment when the patient exhibited other signs of respiratory restriction as well, and at this point, he would recheck these restrictions. Alternatively, perhaps for the same patient, Fulford would approach this problem by placing his thumbs beneath the lower ribs and adding bilateral tension until his fingers gradually sank into the tissue. In addition, if the regional restriction was expressed through fascial connection to the lateral rib cage or as a depression in the right arm, Fulford would address these with local application of the percussion vibrator.

Restrictions of the upper ribs and thorax were treated as a regional unit. The scapula and clavicle were stabilized with one hand while the other grasped the flexed elbow and used the arm as a lever to first rotate the shoulder in a posterior direction, then eventually in a superior direction, completing a circle, as though bringing the patient passively through a throwing motion. (The reader will recognize this as a repetition of the diagnostic sequence discussed in Chapter 7.) The articular technique is a ligamentous stretch with the goal of returning energy to the tissues. If Fulford discovered a restriction and intended to treat it, the added agency of his intention was the critical variable that converted the process of motion testing to that of treatment. He would then recheck the work, saying "Now you can reach into the cookie jar" or "Now you can wave at your girlfriend." He would sometimes complement this maneuver with application of the percussion vibrator to the deltoid region of the shoulder.

If spinal treatments were not performed with direct articular mobilization, they were almost always addressed with percussive vibration or magnets (see Chapter 9).

*Cranial Treatment*

There is no way to succinctly explain what Fulford was doing in the cranium. He did not try to manufacture a hierarchy between the various articular relationships, emphasize a particular aspect of the membranous system, or do anything beyond working with "the energy" reflected in the breath. He would recognize relative immobility of individual bones and sutures. But, as with the remainder of the body, Fulford was of the opinion that the physical body rested in the ethric or energetic body, and that symptoms in the former were reflections of imbalances in the latter. Treatment was directed at the most primary cause. The status and progress of the work were assessed by the intensity and freedom of the breath to affect each moving part. Empirically, this would manifest as a soften-ing, a regional swelling, a warmth, a subtle gliding, and a tactile harmony in the field.

Cranial work was performed in a very special way, blending the induc-tive-intentional mobilization of energy flow with techniques for treating the articular, fluid, and/or membranous relationships. The latter tech-niques are found in more orthodox cranial approaches. Fulford repeated-ly said that the primary mobilizing force was located in the L-field, the bioelectric expression of the person, and not in any aspect of the physical body. Thus, Fulford performed his unique meld of approaches to ensure the proper polarity in the patient.

As noted in Chapter 7, Fulford would approach the cranial area from the front of the body and perform any of a number of techniques (see, e.g., Fig. 8-1):

- He cupped the occipital-temporal area in his palms, that is, he stood to the side and followed the contours of the occiput with one cupped hand, while the other was placed over the frontal bone.

- He used his hand in a cant-hook style to follow the sphenoid anteri-orly and the occiput posteriorly.

- He treated the zygoma and maxillary area by placing his finger pads bilaterally.

In each of these techniques, Fulford was noting the anatomical "excur-sion," but more importantly, he was concerned about palpating the Breath, the fullness of vitality of the field.

*A Divergent View*

Though controversial, it should be related that in preparing for addresses to The Cranial Academy over the last several years of his life, Fulford agonized over how to describe his differences with the majority opinion and still remain a polite gentleman and revered past-president. Among the issues discussed in private conversation was his adamant belief that the cranial rhythmic impulse (CRI) or primary respiratory mechanism

124

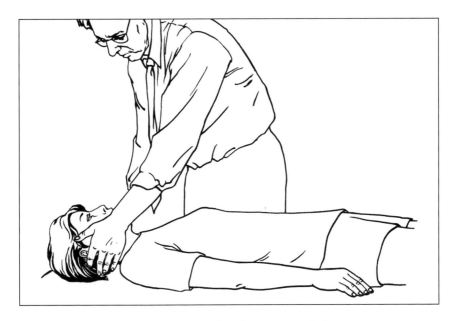

**Fig. 8-1** Anterior approach to the cranium for correct polarity

(PRM) did not exist. On many occasions I tried to convince him to reinterpret the significance of these concepts in his model. Perhaps, I suggested, it was an epiphenomenon, a shadow of a more significant force which Sutherland had described as the Potency. But he would have none of it. He spoke only about the flow of energy, reflected in the Breath, something that was greater than but included involvement of the whole body in filling the lungs.

Although he primarily treated the head while standing or sitting to the side of the patient, I saw Fulford do Sutherland-style articular mobilization that was consistent with the techniques outlined in *Teachings in the Science of Osteopathy*,[4] including treating while seated behind a supine patient. I also saw him treat a patient using only induction of the field: he would concentrate on his sensation of the field, and then direct his intention to use his field to balance the patient's field. If you are trained in osteopathic cranial techniques, you can integrate the techniques and proceed accordingly.

In traditional energy work based on the ideas of South Asian philosophy and medicine, there is a hierarchy of centers (chakras) that traverse the axial part of the body, terminating at the highest center at the top of the head, the crown chakra. Classical cranial osteopathy recognizes an axis of motion that ends anteriorly somewhere near the insertion of the falx cerebri at the crista galli of the ethmoid bone, and the convergence of the tentorium cerebelli with the clinoid processes of the sphenoid. Fulford utilized the idea of an energetic axis, but changed the relationships of the chakra system to accommodate and extend the osteopathic concept.

In the physical body, the most superior part of this axis developmentally proceeds through the nasal and oral area to the precordial area. As described in Chapter 7, the embryological enfolding of the body that moves the heart to its final location in the newborn child carries the pole of the field through this area as well. The sucking reflex, the ability to breathe through the nose, and the fact that the olfactory nerve is an extension of the brain are all a result of this motion. Fulford thought of the zygoma as an accessible prominence, a lever that reflected this relationship and that could be used to induce motion into the anterior cranial area. Fulford found that, prior to his treatment of this area, the flow of breath through it was often inadequate. Following treatment, he would therefore check for a return of the flow of breath to this area. In addition, he would stimulate the philtrum, between the nose and mouth, to reawaken any repressed sucking reflex, especially in children. The continuation of this axis leads to the thymus and heart area in the anterior chest, discussed at length in Chapter 7. Fulford would treat it using the induction technique added to basic cranial mobilization, as mentioned above.

But the body does not end here. The posterior and anterior portions of the body represent a loop of continuous energy flow. It is somewhat like making a snowball, in which you first pat here, then there, and later on the other side, trying to make it round. Working with the field means striving to restore a free-flowing and balanced circuit of energy. You can enter the loop at any point and attend to any aspect that seems helpful in getting the energy to run smoothly. First you work at this end, then at that end, and later a little here and a little there, striving for a harmonious balance. While the sequence described here is important, on a given day Fulford would enter the system of the patient where it suited him.

## A Student's Viewpoint:
## Reflections from the Doctor's Shadow

Dr. Fulford's warm, wise, gentle grin communicated so much. To the patient it seemed to say "I care about you, but be patient. Open your mind and heart and let yourself be led. Life is complex, and you and your body are a process that began long before your birth and will proceed far beyond your death. Let me help you make the most of the moment." And to the student it seemed to say "Try what you see, and try what you know. Integrate but don't parrot what I do. It will come in time."

The purr of the percussion instrument seemed to be an extension of his demeanor and mood: resolute, persistent, strong, and solicitous. The message seemed to be that our desires would bear fruit if they blended with the plan of the Creator. A prayer would carry us further forward than a demand. For after all, the work of the spirit proceeds through our labor, our study, and our commitment to help.

> "What you do for others will eventually return to you. Our emotional lives are connected to those of other people, whether we like it or not. You might want to believe that you're totally independent and that you do and say whatever you wish. The truth is that we all share the same life force, and when you give and re-give to someone else, you're helping your own life force grow."[5]

These are good words to live by.

### REFERENCES

1. Robert Fulford, personal communication, 1989.

2. Sutherland WG. *Teachings in the Science of Osteopathy*. Portland, OR: Rudra Press, 1990.

3. Van Buskirk R. *The Still Technique Manual*. Indianapolis, IN: American Academy of Osteopathy, 1999.

4. Sutherland, *Teachings in the Science of Osteopathy*, 233-84.

5. Fulford's notebooks.

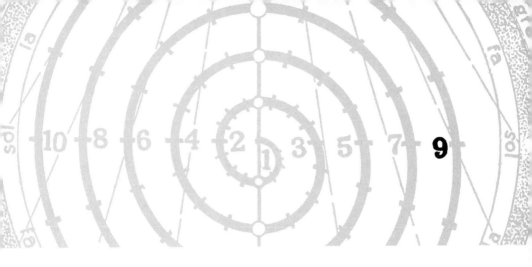

# Adjunctive Modalities

*G*oing through Fulford's drawers and closets was like being given a retrospective view of his life's explorations: there were manuscripts, books, tapes, devices, letters, astrology charts, magnets, homeopathic remedies, and photographs. Looking at the collection and reading his materials made me aware of the breadth of vision of the man and of his resourcefulness as a clinician.

As noted in Chapter 3, Fulford spent much of his early years as a general practitioner. He was refused admission into the military, but was charged with caring for the folks at home. He described long days in the office, a break for supper, back to the office until 8 or 9 in the evening, then home. Often his sleep was interrupted by calls, sometimes requiring home visits. Exhausting! His medical bag from that era included a blood pressure cuff and a stethoscope, but also a panel of homeopathic remedies, including Bach flower remedies.

Fulford explored many different treatment protocols for ways to increase his ability to heal, and also to diminish the cost to him in energy. He explored dietary therapies, astrology, and herbal remedies, but the percussion vibrator and the use of therapeutic crystals and magnets were his mainstays. These therapies will be described in this chapter.

CHAPTER NINE

## Percussion Vibrator: The "Hammer"

In Fulford's closet were small, hand-held vibrators that he had used in his initial attempts to accommodate the vibratory, oscillatory nature of the human being—the energetic body. He told me that, although he was intuitively searching for a device to affect the vibratory life field, none of the early devices had much power. When a pamphlet came in the mail advertising the Foredom Percussion Vibrator, Fulford recalled thinking "That's just what I've been looking for."

The motor he used in his early courses had a large, wire-wrapped armature that hummed with authoritative power and momentum. Over the years, the design and manufacture of the motors changed with advances in technology. However, the Foredom vibrator continued to serve the Doctor's purpose. He consulted with the manufacturer and modifications were made. A receipt in his files showed that he was ordering spare parts from Foredom in 1955. The motor drove a replaceable hand piece by means of a cased flexible shaft. Held in the left hand, it became an extension of that hand, communicating with the monitoring right hand in doing work in the energetic field.

Dr. Fulford was coaxed into presenting his Percussion Vibrator Course in 1986 by Gerry Slattery, a fellow osteopath who thought that his system would be enlightening to other osteopaths. As many have discovered, the tool is a powerful extension of the thought and action of the operator, but it depends for its effectiveness on his or her intention and diagnostic knowledge. It was never presented as a substitute for these essential elements.

Fulford reasoned that trauma in the energetic field resulted in a local lack of resonance, what he called an "energy sink." Building on Still's concept of the importance of the fascia, and the findings of Robert Becker and others regarding the piezoelectric character of tissue, he theorized:

> When a trauma, physical or emotional, takes place in the tissues or bone, a current of injury is created. This results in a depressed area in the tissue. The depression is known as a sink. The sink creates a blockage in the normal flow of the piezoelectric current. It took a force of energy to create the trauma and

130

blockage. In order to correct the blockage to the normal flow, it will require a quantum of energy of the same frequency as the current of injury, but will need a quantum of energy of greater intensity than the current of injury to release the sink. We have found that the percussion vibrator is the instrument of choice.[1]

Fulford would position the oscillating pad perpendicular to the skin surface (Fig. 9-1), inducing resonant oscillations in the tissues and swamping the energy sink with new energy. Fulford believed that this resulted in:

• The return of the natural energy flow

• The entrained return of the endogenous rhythmic character of the tissue.

As he began to work with this tool, he discovered that the work of the "hammer"[2] was really an extension of his intention to intervene. Working in the physical body, it could mobilize restricted tissue, an effect which is

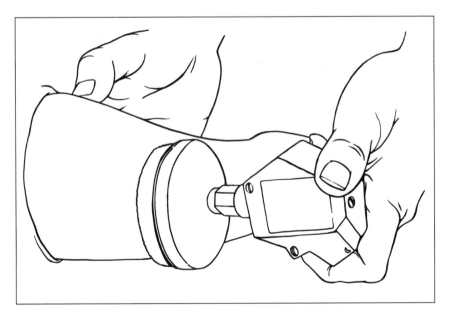

**Fig. 9-1** Demonstration of contact

acknowledged by some osteopaths who utilize this aspect of the tool. However, Fulford came to see that the percussion vibrator had consequences that affected the energetic body as well.

Fulford extended the use of the percussion vibrator to include the treatment of energy centers, reflex associations, and points associated with the birth trauma and/or respiration. In general:

- The pad was applied to bony prominences to spread the vibratory force deep into the tissue along bones and fascial planes (Fig. 9-2).

- The posterior aspect of the body was treated before the anterior aspect (motor before affective).

- The distal parts were usually treated before the proximal parts.

- The hand polarity rules were still followed.

The frequency required to induce resonance varies. Fulford used his monitoring hand to note the distribution, pattern, and degree of resonance. This judgment was also partly based on a sense of the activity of the elec-

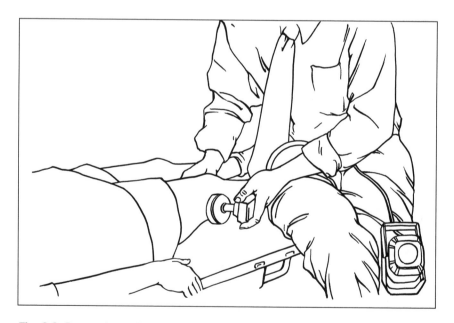

**Fig. 9-2** Percussion to lateral knee

tromagnetic or ethric field, described in Chapter 7. Palpation of the field, and recognition of contours, restriction, and perturbation, can be cultivated with consistent practice. I use the analogy of water, as the feeling on the surface of water provides some sense of field contours: putting your hand in a flow of water gives a hint of the feeling of dynamism in the field. Measuring the frequency also draws on the conventional use in classical osteopathic practice of a motor and monitoring hand. This was amplified by Fulford's approach, which focused on working with triangles—uniting both hands and the attentive mind, as a dialogic unit—to sense the state of the person, and to optimize the release or change of state.

This cannot be adequately explained without actually experiencing the percussion vibrator in a supervised setting. However, if one has a sense for the rhythm and the physical characteristics of tissue, with experience you can develop an expectation of the response to the percussion vibration to be transmitted through a certain amount and type of tissue. A restriction response is perceived as a suboptimal transmission of the applied vibratory force through the physical medium of the tissue. Alternatively, and with more sensitivity, restriction in the ethric body is experienced as a subtle turbulence. The goal of treatment is the return of a harmonic, rhythmic energy flow to the area monitored. An analogy to turbulence and smooth flow of air or water is helpful in guiding concentration during learning.

The Foredom Percussion Vibrator has a range of 0 to 4000 Hz, and the motor force is transmitted by a rotating shaft to a percussive padded hand piece. The stroke amplitude is fixed. To vary the effect, the frequency is changed. The updated version has corrective circuitry to maintain the motor speed under load. Once the percussive vibrator is applied to the tissue, the force pattern creates a response in the tissue that can vary from a dissonant vibration to a harmonic standing wave. A midrange frequency may be a good starting point, but this depends on the density of the tissue and the energized state of the patient. Obviously, because of their different tissue mass, the pelvis would require a higher vibratory rate than the cervical spine.

An initial assessment is made of the qualitative response of the tissue based on the amplitude and quality of the vibration transmitted to the monitoring hand. A release is sensed by a change in the energy field, often corresponding to an audible or palpable vibratory change between the tissue, hand, and motor:

> With the proper speed and positioning of the applicator, the monitoring hand will feel a pulling sensation. This sensation will gradually get a tighter feeling and then a sudden release. The motor will speed up and an awareness of something flowing under the monitoring hand will be felt.[3]

According to Fulford's notes, subtle articular work would often follow the use of percussive vibration. Occasionally, Fulford would apply only local vibration or do a subset of sites after palpating the spinal complex. Distal areas were palpated before proximal sites, partly to deal with:

- The grounding issue raised by Polarity Therapy (see Chapter 7)

- The need to balance the triad of positive, negative, and neutral as reflected in distal, proximal, and midbody tissue, respectively

- Special attention was paid to the anatomic correlates of the energy centers depicted by the chakra system, particularly the coccyx (base chakra), sacrum (second chakra), the thoracolumbar junction (solar plexus), and the midthoracic region (heart chakra).

- We will not describe further the use of the vibrator in the cervical and cranial fields because of the central character of these tissues and the possibility that inexperienced practitioners will inflict significant harm. *These areas should only be approached under supervision of an experienced practitioner.* Let me just say that, in his advanced course, Fulford described the effects to the energy field of the cranial area via percussion to the shoulders and cervical spine, and gentle percussion of selected areas of the cranium. As previously noted, Fulford would be face to face with his patient when doing this work.

With or without the use of a percussion vibrator, Fulford would work with:

- Concentration

- Focused intention

- Union with the patient

- An intent to serve

- An invocation for help from the Creative Force.

Although there were guidelines for doing this work, all of his actions were guided by what he felt in the experiential event with the patient.

Percussor work did not constitute a general treatment. Rather, it was tied closely to the diagnostic findings. As Fulford wrote:

> In using the percussion vibrator, one must with your mind establish an 'element of specific intent.' You have located the blockage in the muscle, joint, or bone by determining the malalignment of the area involved.[4]

Percussion can be applied to a site of past focal trauma, for example, the cervico-occipital area or the left shoulder. However, the lumbar and sacral areas received special attention because of the frequency of restrictions. With the patient lying in the supine position, the percussion vibrator in the practitioner's left hand, and the monitoring hand on the left iliac area, percussion was applied to the right trochanter (Fig. 9-3). The oscillatory response monitored by the right hand was used in making adjustments to the frequency of the percussive vibrator, the pressure placed on the tissue, and the duration of the treatment. This was done until the tissue responded appropriately, signaling the presence of spontaneous resonance in the test region.

Next, with the patient in a lateral recumbent position, the percussion vibrator in the practitioner's left hand, the monitoring right hand on the uppermost iliac crest, Fulford would percuss the spine from the sacrum upward (Fig. 9-4). When the vibrator reached the midlumbar area, he would sometimes move his monitoring hand to the periumbilical area. Fulford felt a connection between the motility of the gut (presently and in the process of fetal development) and the lumbar spine.[5] Above the

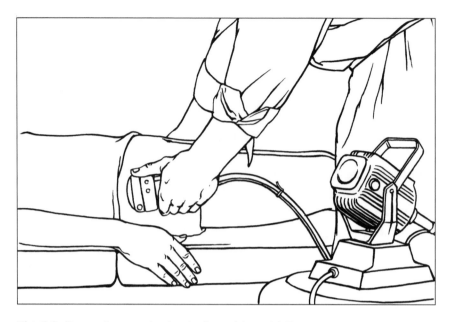

**Fig. 9-3** Percussion over trochanter for pelvic restriction

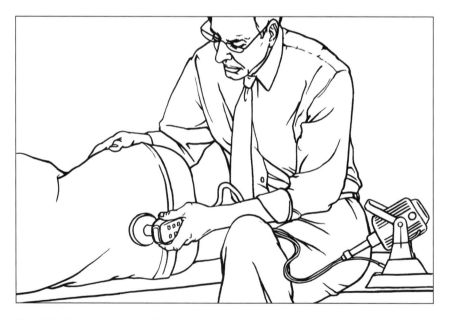

**Fig. 9-4** Percussion to lumbar spine and sacrum

thoracolumbar junction, the monitoring hand was moved to the upper-most shoulder (Fig. 9-5).

Throughout this work, Fulford was assessing tissue response, respiratory response, and the ethric field to determine changes in the restriction. Generally, a change will occur in the three parameters concurrently. Individual regions will vary in their response. With practice, the physician can learn to distinguish between differences that simply reflect variation in tissue density as a result of regional anatomy, and those that represent functional changes or changes in the field.

Fulford gave special attention to certain regions because of their association with patterns, for example, with the birth process, or with Stone's companion vertebrae. The occiput, the shoulders (especially the left one), and the left knee were prone to restriction because of their role in the most common birth presentation of left-occiput-anterior (see Chapter 4). Fulford also used information concerning *in utero* conditions in his treatment. For example, when he treated the left knee, he would sometimes

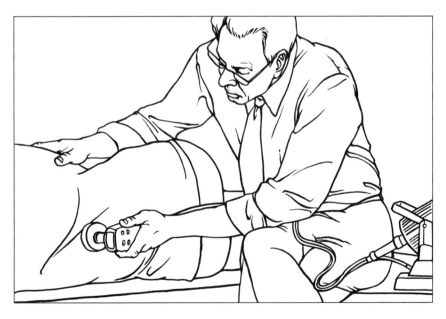

**Fig. 9-5** Percussion to thoracolumbar spine

flex this knee and place the sole of the foot against the medial right knee. He felt that there was a more effective flow of energy in this position, possibly because this limb position is common *in utero*.[6]

In Chapter 5 we noted the association of emotional and physical factors with the diaphragm, the heart chakra, and the solar plexus, all of which Fulford sometimes termed the *visceral brain*. If the target of the treatment session were emotional release, Fulford would percuss the posterior or motor side of the midthoracic area (T4 especially) before applying vibratory force over the sternal area. (The T4 area will return in our discussion of crystals.) Again, the practitioner should recognize that this area of work exists, but, for the safety of the healer and patient, should not proceed without guided instruction.

No rules were ever really finalized, and Fulford never wrote up the description of his treatments for publication. He felt that he was still exploring, changing, and adding. He taught his courses from his notebooks, which he guarded. He was always reading, reflecting, revising, and adding notes in the margin.

## Crystals

Fulford developed his use of quartz crystals as a result of the work of Marcel Vogel (1917–1991). French Canadian and Catholic born, Vogel had a near-death illness in childhood that later prevented his full participation in formal higher education. However, he taught himself chemistry, and developed a special interest in biophosphorescence. As a young man, his work as a sign painter included the use of fluorescent paints. Eventually, he became a scientist with IBM and was involved in the early work with fluorescent lighting and the magnetic coatings on computer hard drives.

Later in his career, Vogel attempted to measure the emotional response of plants to language, which had been propounded by Cleve Baxter, and described by others.[7] Vogel was initially skeptical of this claim, but, with the use of a simple voltmeter—somewhat akin to a polygraph machine—he noted a measurable electrical response to injury or threat of injury in plants. Vogel subsequently discovered that plants were sensitive not only to our actions, but also to our words and thoughts, and that this response could be amplified by a refined cut quartz crystal in conjunction with thoughts that were timed to the individual's breath.[8]

After years of refinement, Vogel extended this work to humans. He established a retreat and training center for further study of these phenomena. To intensify the effect, he found a way to modify the facet angles of the crystals, guided by the molecular pattern of water. Using precision cutting that was guided by the absorption spectra of the transmitted light beam, he standardized the crystal designs. In the end, his protocol included:

- Mutual acceptance between the healer and subject. This means that the disposition of the healer must be one of empathetic acceptance. Unconditional love would be a more emphatic way of describing Vogel's approach, upon which Fulford modeled some of his own method. Reciprocally, the patient obtained maximal benefit if he or she were trusting in their attitude toward the physician, and accepting of change.

- Awareness of every aspect of the treatment, including the emotional aspect

- Invocation of the help of the Creator

- Having a loving intention to heal

- Acceptance by the patient of subsequent follow-up work.

The crystal, charged with the *pulsed breath* as well as the healer's loving intention and prayers, amplified the intention for maximal effect. The pulsed breath is a way of maximizing the operator's intention through use of the breath on the crystal. The forced nasal exhalation sounds like a mild snort. This is performed once on each face or side of the crystal, to cleanse and charge it.

Fulford visited Vogel and incorporated his concepts and the use of crystals in his work, as he felt it was compatible with his way of healing.

In his last presentation to the osteopathic community (see Appendix B), he demonstrated a variation of his technique called the Ring of Fire, named after a protocol described by Norman Shealy and Carolyn Myss.[9] The crystal works directly in the energy field (L-field, ethric body) of the person. It requires that the practitioner first cultivate a sensitivity for feeling the qualitative and quantitative variations within each patient and between patients. This skill does not come easily. Clear, refined, cut quartz crystal is used to energize, while a smoky quartz crystal is used to extract energy.

The point of physical contact for the emotional body is located superior to the thymus, or anterior sternum, which in turn corresponds to the heart center. Fulford sometimes referred to this as the anterior counterpart to the T4 dorsal segment. The significance of this segment was an empirical observation of Fulford's. There is a viscerosomatic relationship between this area and the heart reported in conventional osteopathic literature.[10] Fulford also used crystals to treat specific sites of pain, especially if there were a focal perturbation in the field. According to Vogel,[11] several protocols may be used, including:

- The crystal can be cradled between the thumb, index and middle fingers, using the more acute angle as the pointer.

- The healer can rub the crystal with the thumb until it is felt to be alive. It is then charged and cleared with a pulsed breath directed toward each flat side.

- Most commonly, the area to be treated is approached with the acute end of the crystal. The point is directed in a counterclockwise circle to enter the field. Once the feeling of opening or penetration has occurred, the practitioner uses a reciprocating linear motion to sweep and engage the field, thereby starting the work.

- The sweeping motions can be performed like a circling pendulum until the practitioner feels maximum engagement, that is, a sense of engagement, turbulence, or resistance. At this point, the sweeping motions are continued until a feeling of release, harmony, or peacefulness is obtained. By reversing the circular motion in a clockwise direction, the practitioner can close and leave the field.

Much of this will be clearer to those who have experience with subtle motion testing, assessing slight resistance, and sensing the tide and potency of cranial manipulation. This was the doorway through which Dr. Fulford entered, especially considering his work with Sutherland. As noted in Chapter 4, in the 1940s Fulford and Sutherland conducted experiments to determine the effect of oscillatory motion and light on the energy models of Walter Russell. He was already exposed to the idea of a life field. One wonders how much success in this work is dependent on intuition, individual talent, or invitation.

## Magnets

The first time I asked Dr. Fulford to work on a patient for whom my treatment had failed happened to be my wife. We were at the 1991 AAO Convocation in Kansas City, and since I wanted to learn more about Fulford's work, I asked him to treat her. He invited us to his hotel room after the meetings were finished. I felt too foolish to bring my percussion vibrator, which I had enthusiastically brought along on the trip. I left it packed. Fulford was wise and powerful enough not to need his. After we both assessed the patient, lying prone on the bed, and agreed on the poor state of her midthoracic spine and ribs, he prepared to work. Dr. Fulford went to the wardrobe and removed a pair of magnets, about 10 x 25 cm in size, separated them, and placed one on each side of the spinal column at the level of dysfunction. He closed his eyes, concentrated, and waited. After removing the magnets, we both reevaluated the patient and found the tissue to be relaxed and symmetric.

This was the typical protocol for his use of magnets. He did not use them often, and the ones he chose are available from a popular electronics supply company. They had a power of approximately 500 gauss and were sold as audio speaker magnets. On several occasions we discussed the popular trend of using magnets in shoe insoles, mattresses, and clothing. This, in his view, represented a risk of overexposure by an unregulated dose on an undiagnosed condition with unknown effect. As far as the ethric body was concerned, the effect might be innocuous, successful, or harmful. Magnetic devices represented a potent force that, to work correctly, needed to be applied judiciously and under supervision; but most importantly, they needed the facilitating intention of the diagnosing and treating practitioner. The success and power of magnets lay in the interpersonal interaction, and not merely in some innate property of the magnets.

## Other Modalities

The Doctor went through many phases in his practice during which he would investigate, integrate, and refine the use of a number of modalities. He attended to nutrition, but in the end he paid attention to the natural quality of the food. He went through a period of astrological charting, which for him involved a large amount of detail. By the time I met him, this was only in his resource pile. He had used homeopathic and Bach flower remedies, and still used Rescue Remedy. He continued to use herbals as prescribed by practitioners using muscle testing of the opponens pollicis muscle derived from applied kinesiology. I have had some exposure to these and other modalities, but because of their limited use in Fulford's later synthesis, and my own limited ability in integrate them, I have chosen not to describe them here. Let me simply say that Dr. Fulford expected us to be guided by intuition in our use of anything that was honestly helpful and put in our path. He used conventional medication and hospital care, and saw no philosophical conflict with this. However, he also sought help from me when treatment according to his own principles seemed preferable to conventional medical care.

REFERENCES

1. Robert Fulford, course notebook (unpublished), page 12.

2. Fulford used this word for years because of the power of the device, but he later dropped it for liability reasons, and for its negative nuances when advertising the course.

3. Robert Fulford, course notebook (unpublished), page 24.

4. Ibid., 23.

5. Robert Fulford, personal communication.

6. Cunningham FG et al. (eds.) *Williams Obstetrics*, 20th ed. Stamford, CT: Appleton and Lang, 1997: 319.

7. Tompkins T. *The Secret Life of Plants.* New York: Avon, 1974.

8. Vogel M. Miscellaneous tapes and newsletters from Psychic Research, Inc., San Jose, CA (now closed). Check availability through Lifestream Associates, 70 Sable Court, Winter Springs, FL 32708.

9. Shealy CN, Myss C. The ring of fire and dhea: a theory for restoration of adrenal reserves. *Subtle Energies* 6(2):167-75.

10. Ward R. *Foundations of Osteopathic Medicine.* Baltimore: Williams and Wilkins, 1997: 571.

11. As previously noted, these course handouts were originally published by the now defunct Institute of Psychic Research.

PART FOUR

# Future Directions for Medicine

"We have given a few thoughts on this line of life, hoping
the osteopath will take up the subject and travel a few
miles farther toward the fountain of this great source of
knowledge and apply the results to the relief and comfort
of the afflicted who come for counsel and advice."

—*Andrew Taylor Still*

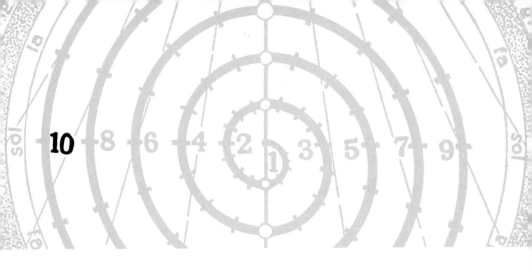

# An Expanded Osteopathic Concept: Keeping Up with Progressive Medicine and Science

### A Sometimes Problematic Approach

To those who have not personally experienced their effectiveness, Dr. Fulford's methods may seem strange. Just as William Sutherland's methods, in the early days of cranial osteopathy, were thought to be unacceptably different, so too has Fulford's approach often been difficult to reconcile with other osteopathic methods. Yet, rather than trying to justify his approach, Fulford chose instead to ignore the criticism and to simply "dig on" through more reading, experimentation, observation, and treatment.

One of my motivations for taking a position at an osteopathic school was to have time to read and do research in areas of physiology and osteopathic principles, and to make linkages to Fulford's concepts and methods. Like other original thinkers before him, Fulford's work makes more sense in the context of a diverse frontier of knowledge which is moving toward a new integrated synthesis. This chapter reflects some of my thoughts regarding the compatibility of Fulford's methods with other osteopathic approaches, and how they contribute to a better understanding of fundamental questions of human health.

CHAPTER TEN

# The Complementarity of Different Models

Many of the ideas enunciated by Dr. Fulford, for example, the idea that the ethric body is part of the causal chain responsible for the symptoms and palpable dysfunctions seen in patients, seem at first glance to be unrelated to the conventional osteopathic understanding of the interrelationship between structure and function. However, recall that A.T. Still, the founder of osteopathy, stressed the integral unity of the person in making all physical diagnosis. He was quite open-ended about what that meant. In his own day, Still's association with Spiritualism and his thoughts on the biogenic life force presented a challenge to his family and students.[1]

Others have expanded osteopathic thought in this direction. As early as 1906, a brief work entitled *Esoteric Osteopathy*[2] suggested that the osteopathic approach should include the Hindu transcendental view of the person. Later, in the early to mid-twentieth century, some of Sutherland's concepts, for example, the primary respiratory mechanism and cranial articular motion, presented challenges to the osteopathic community and served as catalysts for growth.

In the 1930s, Charlotte Weaver related the shape and function of the cranium to evolutionary embryology, stating that the tripartite brain had evolved to regulate the body's participation with vibratory energies, or ether waves, in addition to chemical energies in the conventional biochemical sense. She recognized a pattern of mobile segments in the cranium which corresponded to a pattern of interaction between developmental ossification centers and mature bones of the cranial base.[3]

More recently, other leaders in osteopathy, such as Viola Frymann, have suggested that an expanded osteopathic concept based on a fuller appreciation of the cranial mechanism through research represents the osteopathy of the future.[4] Indeed, several scientists have made inroads in this important area. For example, Yuri Moskalenko, working with Frymann, focused on measuring patterns of interaction between intracranial volume and pressure changes, which he associates with defined dysfunction before and after cranial treatment.[5]

Others are taking things in slightly different directions. Kenneth Nelson and his colleagues recently reconceptualized the cranial rhythm as the composite Traube Herring wave, a recognized and measurable medical phenomenon.[6] Douglas Richards and others demonstrated the vascular response to manipulation of the vasomotor center.[7] James Jealous remodeled cranial osteopathy along the lines of the "Long Tide."[8] And Judith O'Connell has pursued the deeper significance of connective tissue work.[9]

Fulford's diagnostic and treatment methods likewise offer a new challenge to our guiding principles and a new way of defining the person. Consider, for example, his claim that pain, strain, and trauma have an energetic and emotional component, in addition to the physical component, that can be manipulated.

## Definition of Treatment Goals in Various Models

Dr. Still repeatedly challenged us to base our practice on our understanding of the whole person. He encouraged his students to look for a primary cause in the anatomy of a patient. Anatomy was primary.[10] Yet at the same time he emphasized the person's triunal nature: physical, spiritual, and mental.[11] The spiritual side of the person can be attributed to the fact that the body was created by a superior intelligence, God, who he referred to as the Great Architect.[12] Herein lies a dilemma that the children of Still must face: how to deal with both the physical anatomy as well as the other dimensions of the human being.

The early osteopathic literature used the construct of the *osteopathic lesion* to explain the cause of symptoms. Later this term was replaced with *somatic dysfunction*. Each of these terms has been defined in a variety of ways, with each definition emphasizing selected aspects of a causal network of physical interactions in the body. In these models, the interrelationship of structure and function has been postulated to revolve around such features as:

- articular integrity and position[13]

- ligamentous laxity[14]

- neuromuscular reflexes, including facilitation[15]

- imbalances in gamma motor neuron modulation[16]

- respiratory restriction and tissue fluid stasis[17]

- unbalanced fascial tension[18]

- stress bands resulting from trauma[19]

- mood alteration secondary to trauma and stress.[20]

Some of these are considered to be primary factors, others secondary in nature. The proponents of each method believe that the integrated dynamics of regions and of the whole body are altered in response to changes in these factors.

## The Future

I would suggest that the future of osteopathy lies in recognizing the value of the expansive, sensitive observation of one hundred-plus years of osteopathic investigation, and with an appreciation of the various facets that make the body a self-regulating and functional unit.[21] In defining function and dysfunction, Fulford emphasized the electromagnetic character of the body, its movement patterns, and the influences upon it. Although others before him had promulgated the idea of "oscillatory intervention," the target was a mechanically defined dysfunction.[22] Fulford's shift in emphasis altered the way palpation and manipulation were to be conducted, and made the practitioner focus on more subtle relationships.

There is a measure of validity in each of these approaches, be they articulated by Fryette, Korr, Mitchell, or Fulford. The key to a successful practice is to know when to emphasize the particular element that contributes to the integration of structure and function. Or, as Still admonished us:

> Every operator should use his own judgment and choose his own method of adjusting all the bones of the body. It is not a matter of imitation and doing

just as some successful operator does, but the bringing of the bone from the
abnormal to the normal.[23]

The particular method should be based on the nature of the patient and
the problem. However, it is also based on the physician's treatment
approach and the way he or she selects certain empirical, and deduced,
criteria to structure a diagnosis from the findings. For example, those who
appreciate:

- the *thrust or muscle energy approach* can concentrate on the relative vertebral resistance to motion, sometimes represented by asymmetric
  positional displacement.[24]

- a *ligamentous tension release approach* would explore periarticular ligamentous laxity and restriction.[25]

- *functional methods* can explore the degree of ease and bind in these segments and would describe the sense of ease in the total tissue while
  postulating the effect of a neural pattern generator on maintaining the
  asymmetry.[26]

- the *nociceptive model* would suggest that the biomechanics of the pain
  process maintain the abnormal body position, complementing the
  older concept of sympathetically modulated facilitation.[27]

- the *counterstrain approach* would be guided by the patient's history and
  point of tenderness to deduce the position of ease; they would then
  confirm their conclusions by positioning the body in a way that the
  point of tenderness disappears, postulating that the strain was a result
  of an imbalance in the gamma motor neuron input to muscle spin-
  dles.[28]

- a *connective approach* would attribute the dysfunction to regional relationships involving freedom or restriction of fascia and ligaments,
  perhaps considering their bioelectromechanical qualities as well.[29]

In addition to these methods, cranial-based approaches have their own
expanded constellation of data points to consider when formulating a

diagnosis and a planned intervention, all the while still working with the same body. In this vein, Fulford's method of inquiry included the extended use of the same contacts, tissue texture analyses, and motion tests, but with a twist. Each of these models deals with asymmetric ease and binding in the tissue. Fulford simply added another level of interaction between the patient and physician, one that we need to cultivate, just as we worked on developing our "tissue sense" in our initial weeks of osteopathic college. We must learn to palpate the subtle body.

## Recent Data

### Interpersonal Physical Effects

One way of looking at this is that the nonphysical contact is just plain unscientific, and that Fulford's sources are more than a little dated. However, part of the medical community has a different perspective. Bolstered by the less commonly used aspects of physics (though not totally neglected in this age of lasers, PET scans, and high emission radiation treatment), physicians such as Larry Dossey, author of *Healing Words*,[30] *Prayer is Good Medicine*,[31] and *Reinventing Medicine*,[32] have summarized the data for interpersonal physical effects from healers, nonlocal physical effect experiments, and "retroactive" physical effects. An example of the latter are studies[33] noted by Dossey of the effects of intercessory prayer by participants blinded to growth rates of bacteria during a prior time interval. In these experiments growth rates of bacteria on two groups of agar plates were compared. The plates for which prayers were said for better growth showed faster growth. The data are cited in Dossey's work as supportive of the ideas of the potential physical effect of intention in healing, and of the emotional impact of trauma.

### Hebb's Notion of Patterns of Discharge

Osteopathy has shown a great interest in the coordinative function of the nervous system, from Still's focus on nerve force, to Korr and Denslow's work with facilitation, to Frank Willard's explanation of pain pathways and interneuronal communication. I would suggest that there are still other ways to envision the nervous system. In our experiments, we explore the various levels of interaction between the central nervous system, peripheral nervous system, and neuromuscular junction, and the effect of outside influences on this pathway, including reflex loops, potentiation, and inhibition. From Donald Hebb's work in the 1940s,[34, 35] there has arisen in neurology another line of thought concerning the structure and function of the nervous system. According to Hebb, actions are initiated not just by the quantified summation of depolarization potentials reaching a threshold for depolarization at the postsynaptic membranes in the pathway. Rather, the precipitating event within the afferent and efferent sides of a circuit may be governed not by the quantity of discharge, but by patterns of discharge. In other words, many processes involve depolarization and repolarization cycles. The frequency or pattern of *cyclic* discharge constitutes a code for operating or activating in the system. Physicians are very familiar with this mode of operation in cardiac physiology.

Many neurophysiologists are recognizing that the manner of coding visual (and probably many other) stimuli in the brain as memory involves the rate and pattern of resonant depolarization of cells, so called *resonant cell assemblies*.[36] This mechanism, where special interneuronal coordination is replaced by temporal and spatial patterning of communication, is not hampered by the "coding and binding problem," which answers the question: How does the brain record, interpret, and selectively respond to stimuli? This mechanism (resonant cell assemblies[37]) overcomes the classical problem of whether there is sufficient physical space and neurons in the brain to dedicate specific circuits to each thought, sensation, or memory. Rather, this model (dedicated neurons) is replaced by patterns of cell depolarization, that is, spatial and temporal patterns, in which each neuron may participate in many patterns or events. Recurrent depolarizations in one pattern dominate until replaced by a newly initiated, stronger pattern.

These concepts, when extended to the peripheral nervous system, form the neural basis for understanding function and dysfunction. The nervous systems of many animals and of humans is now under scrutiny to unravel the mechanism of the pattern generators that govern, for example, end tissue activation in muscle.[38, 39, 40] In a work by Kelso,[41] the relevance of dynamic patterns of organization in biological processes has been exquisitely modeled, using concepts from chaos theory to describe many phenomena of nature. The theories of attractor functions and cusp shifts in patterns provide a conceptual model for the relationship between functional states (normal function and dysfunction), the generic concept of central pattern generation, and, in particular, the relationship of competing resonant cell assembly patterns in response to successive stimuli.

In the practical application of this theory, one muscle physiologist, Giseller Schalow, has proposed that in the peripheral nervous system—the area of interest to osteopaths—there is constant rhythmic depolarization of muscle in a very fine pattern, subliminal to the patterns seen on routine EMGs. Rather, the activity of cooperating fibers in a gross muscle, the coordinated activity of bilateral agonists, and the reflex activity of contralateral antagonists are coordinated by phase synchrony or phase changes in functionally linked muscle fibers. In his experimental work on rehabilitating patients with partial spinal cord transections, Schalow has shown that oscillatory percussion through mechanically assisted stepping or bouncing by the patient facilitates the return of normal muscle activity.[42] In lay terms, the language for communication within the community of motor neurons involved in both voluntary and classical reflexes is *patterns* of rhythmic depolarization. I would suggest that these results are intriguingly compatible with Fulford's statement at the convocation that all motion is rhythmic motion (see Appendix C).

My current line of work is building on these insights. There is a commonly known, but less frequently investigated, phenomenon in neurophysiology called the *tonic vibratory reflex*. This is distinct from the Hoffman, or H reflex, and the stretch reflexes, and can be demonstrated in animal models. When a vibratory stimulus of the correct frequency is applied over the body of a muscle, the gamma proprioceptive input is changed so that position sense in the limb is lost and there may be in its place an illusion of movement, thereby altering the motor response. Somehow the percussive vibration alters the function of the complex, multicomponent proprioceptive controls that maintain baseline muscle tone.[43]

Could Fulford's application of a percussion vibrator be intervening at the proprioceptive level intended by other better-known osteopathic methods, for example, the functional method, counterstrain method, or muscle energy method? Can vibrations entrain endogenous rhythms within muscles that restore phasic balance? Studies are currently underway to look at this relationship. Additionally, a manual means of inputting therapeutic oscillatory force, called Facilitated Oscillatory Release, is also being developed and tested by the author.[44]

Although inaccurate in detail, many of Still's speculations about the nature of the body were revolutionary prophesies of the scientific knowledge to come. I see Fulford's insights into the practical application of intention and electromagnetic force in the same light. Why should it be so surprising to osteopaths that there is an electromechanical dimension to the musculoskeletal work that we do? Scientists are using the relevant electromagnetic characteristics of tissue to design appropriate diagnostic and treatment tools, for example, MRI, PET scans, and laser surgery. Fulford's work simply encourages us to use our hands as transducers, and our hearts and minds as the central processing units for data.

Attending continuing education courses and seminars, reviewing new publications, listening on the Web, and perusing Fulford's piles of fan mail, one is reinforced in the idea that this man was a pillar of strength, a beacon of insight, and a genuine conduit for healing. How will we follow him to serve others and further shape the destiny of our work?

## REFERENCES

1. Trowbridge C. *Andrew Taylor Still, 1828-1917.* Kirksville, MO: The Thomas Jefferson University Press, 1991: 106-11, 196.

2. Hoffman H. *Esoteric Osteopathy.* Philadelphia: self-published, 1908.

3. Weaver C. The primary brain vesicles and the three cranial vertebra. *JAOA* 1938;37(8):348.

4. Viola Frymann, *2000 International Symposium on Traditional Osteopathy.*

5. Moskalenko Y. "Principles of Instrumental Measurement of the Efficacy of Osteopathy in the Cranial Field." Speech given at the 1999 Symposium of the Deutsche Osteopathie Kolleg.

6. Sergueef N, Nekson K, Glonek T. Changes in the traube-herring wave following cranial manipulation. *AAO Journal* 2001;11(1):17-19.

7. Richards D, McMillin D, Mein E, Nelspon C. Osteopathic regulation of physiology. *AAO Journal* 2000;11(3):34-8.

8. Jealous J. *Emergence of Originality: A Biodynamic View of Osteopathy in the Cranial Field.* Franconia, NH: self-published (no date provided).

9. O'Connell, J. *Bioelectric Fascial Activation and Release.* Indianapolis, IN: American Academy of Osteopathy, 2000.

10. Still AT. *Philosophy of Osteopathy.* Colorado Springs, CO: American Academy of Osteopathy, 1946 (orig. 1899): 16.

11. Ibid., 26.

12. Still AT. *Autobiography of A.T. Still.* Indianapolis, IN: American Academy of Osteopathy, 1981 (orig. 1908): 330.

13. Fryette H. *Principles of Osteopathic Technique.* Indianapolis, IN: American Academy of Osteopathy, 1994 (orig. 1954); Littlejohn JM. *The Fundamentals of Osteopathic Technique,* Maidstone, England: Institute of Classical Osteopathy, 1975; Maigne R. *Diagnosis and Treatment of Pain of Vertebral Origin.* Baltimore: Williams and Wilkins, 1996.

14. Dorman T. *Prolotherapy in the Lumbar Spine and Pelvis.* Philadelphia: Hanley and Belfus, 1995.

15. Korr I. *The Collected Papers of Irvin M. Korr.* Indianapolis, IN: American Academy of Osteopathy, 1979; Patterson M. A model mechanism for spinal segmental facilitation. *JAOA* 1976;76:62-72.

16. Mitchell F. *The Muscle Energy Manual,* vol. 1. East Lansing, MI: MET Press, 1995.

17. Zink JG. Respiratory and circulatory care, the conceptual model. *Osteopathic Annals* 1977;5(3):108-12.

18. Chila A. "Fascial-ligamentous Release." In *Foundations for Osteoapthic Medicine,* Ward R (ed.) Baltimore: Williams and Wilkins, 1997: 819.

19. Typaldos S. *Orthopathic Medicine: The Unification of Orthopedics and Osteopathy through the Fascial Distortion Model.* Brewer, ME: Orthopathic Global Press, 1997.

20. Fulford R. *Dr. Fulford's Touch of Life.* New York: Pocket Books, 1996.

21. Still AT. *Osteopathy Research and Practice.* Seattle: Eastland Press, 1992 (orig. 1910): 9; Still, *Philosophy of Osteopathy,* 40.

22. Comeaux Z. The role of vibration and oscillation in the development of osteopathic thought. *AAO Journal* 2000;10(3):19–24.

23. Still, *Osteopathy Research and Practice*, 21.

24. Kappler R. in *Foundations for Osteopathic Medicine*. Baltimore: Williams and Wilkins, 1997: 667; Mitchell F. *The Muscle Energy Manual*, vol. 1. East Lansing, MI: MET Press, 1995.

25. Chila A. in *Foundations for Osteopathic Medicine*, 819.

26. Johnston W. *Functional Methods*. Indianapolis, IN: American Academy of Osteopathy, 1994: 2-4.

27. Van Buskirk R. Nociceptive reflex and somatic dysfunction, a model. *JAOA*, 1990;90(9):792; Korr I. *The Collected Papers of Irvin M. Korr*. Indianapolis, IN: American Academy of Osteopathy, 1979; Patterson M. A model mechanism for spinal segmental facilitation. *JAOA* 1976;76:62-72.

28. Jones L. *Jones Strain CounterStrain*, 2nd ed. Boise, ID: Jones Strain-CounterStrain Inc., 1995: 13-15.

29. Friedman H, Gilliar W, Glassman J. *Myofascial and Fascial-ligamentous Approaches in Osteopathic Manipulative Medicine*. San Francisco: San Francisco International Manual Medicine Society, 2000.

30. Dossey L. *Healing Words*. New York: Harper Collins, 1993.

31. Dossey L. *Prayer is Good Medicine*. San Francisco: Harper, 1996.

32. Dossey L. *Reinventing Medicine: Beyond Mind-Body to the New Era of Healing*. San Francisco: Harper, 1999.

33. Nash C. Psychometric control of bacterial mutation. *Journal of American Society of Psychical Research* 1984:78(2):145-52.

34. Hebb D. *The Organization of Behavior*. New York: Wiley, 1942.

35. Miguel A. Hebb's dream: the resurgence of cell assemblies. *Neuron* 1997;19:219–22.

36. Hebb, *The Organization of Behavior*; Miguel, Hebb's dream, 219-21.

37. Varela FJ. Resonant cell assemblies: a new approach to cognitive functions and neuronal synchrony. *Biological Research* 1995;28(1):81-95.

38. Spatz H. Hebb's concept of synaptic plasticity and neuronal cell assemblies. *Behavior Brain Research* 1996;78(1):3–7.

39. Samsonvich A, McNaughton B. Path propagation and cognitive mapping in a continuous attractor neural network model. *Journal Neuroscience* 1997;17(15):5900–920.

40. Sakumarai Y. Population coding of cell assemblies—what is in the brain? *Neuroscience Research* 1996;26(1):1-16.

41. Kelso JA. *Dynamic Patterns: The Self-Organization of Brain and Behavior.* Cambridge, MA: MIT Press, 1995.

42. Schalow G, Zach G. Neuronal reorganization through oscillator formation training in patients with cns lesions. *Journal of Peripheral Nervous System* 1998;3:165-88.

43. Eklund G, Hagbarth K. Normal variability of tonic vibration reflexes in man. *Experimental Neurology* 1966;16:80-92; Roll JP, Gilhodes JC. Proprioceptive sensory codes mediating movement trajectory perception: human hand vibration-induced drawing illusions. *Canadian Journal of Physiology and Pharmacology* 1995;73:295-304.

44. Comeaux Z. Facilitated oscillatory release—a method of dynamic assessment and treatment of somatic dysfunction. *AAO Journal,* in press.

APPENDIX A

# Core Statement

The human body is composed of complex streams of moving
energy. When these energy streams become blocked or con-
stricted, we lose the physical, emotional, and mental fluidity
potentially available to us. If the blockage lasts long enough,
the result is pain, discomfort, illness, and distress.

*—Robert C. Fulford, D.O.*

While engaged in reading, Fulford would constantly write lists of factors
to consider, drawing pictures of the conceptual relationships between
ideas or active principles, and writing aphorisms. These filled many notebooks. In the same spirit, he prepared this statement as part of his presentation at the 1992 Convocation of the American Academy of Osteopathy, where he had the opportunity to present his ideas on the theme of
vibratory energy. He said that this statement represented the kernel of his
ideas, a creed of his beliefs about practice. He prepared a poster with this
message, in large type, which he displayed on the wall of his office, and
which he brought along to his courses.

# Fulford's Final Presentation to the Profession: Day One

The following reflects an earnest effort to record Fulford's final public appearance at the June, 1997 Cranial Academy Convention, which took place in Chicago. The material here is drawn from notes made by the author during and immediately after Fulford's talks. This appendix summarizes the material covered in his talk on the first day, with an emphasis on theory. Appendix C covers the material discussed on the second day, with an emphasis on some of his latest methods of treatment.

## Attending the Meeting

For several winters, Dr. Fulford had heart failure, but a combination of physical and energetic medicine allowed him to attend the meeting in the summer of 1997. Carol Dawson arrived in Chicago a week in advance to make things as comfortable for him as possible. Richard Koss, as usual, assisted him in many ways.[1]

I ran errands and was otherwise supportive. Madeline Rathjen, his previous office assistant and companion, was there, as were Sarah Saxton and Paula Eschtruth. These individuals helped make his attendance at this meeting possible, and helped him maintain his wonderful demeanor. Attending this meeting was important to Dr. Fulford for both personal and professional reasons, as was evident in his glee at being able to play with a child in the lobby while waiting for the elevator.

## Speaking on the Chronic Effects of Trauma

On the first day of the conference, Dr. Fulford addressed the assembly of The Cranial Academy Convention. He said that he had been in the hospital four times in the past eight months, and thus his talk had never got written. He would speak "off the top of his head." He said that he regretted for a number of years that he did not make a full intellectual disclosure of his thoughts at a Cranial Academy event.

Fulford related some of his personal history: his birth in 1905 in Cincinnati, Ohio; graduation from the Kansas City School in 1941; meeting with William Sutherland in 1939, and then studying with him in 1942, and later with Beryl Arbuckle in 1953. From the film presented during this talk (discussed at length below), we learned about Fulford's early years of practice. During World War II, he was not called into military service, which allowed him to use his medical skills as a physician at home.

He said that he considered himself a "renegade":

> I guess I may be considered an oddball by The Cranial Academy, since I never quite gave agreement with everything that has been said. I had been associating with MDs, did experiments, and my eyes had been opened.

Fulford did not think of himself as part of the osteopathic mainstream. He attributed this to several things: his approach to the body as a whole, his rationale for placing a hold on the head, and his disagreement about the cranial rhythmic impulse, which he claimed did not exist.[2]

Fulford recalled Sutherland discussing the primary respiratory mechanism (as distinct from the secondary pulmonary respiration) and the five motions of the cranium. Fulford noted that the primary respiration was

162

vital to the patient, and that it can be restricted during birth or as a result of early trauma, including emotional trauma.

Problems here may present themselves at age three or four as learning disabilities, at age 27 or 30 as emotional problems, or later in life as arthritis or impaired vision or hearing. He went on to describe the motion of the fascia and its function in lymphatic drainage and the health of the ear.

Fulford proposed that good diagnosis involved looking at the quality of the respiratory motion. Good respiration included more rib cage motion and not so much abdominal breathing, as well as good excursion of the diaphragm. The diagnosis should also involve checking the skull's contour.

He described how, in the mid-1980s, Dr. Andrew Weil had come to his office to learn more about the percussion vibrator. Expecting to stay no more than an hour, he arrived at one and left at four-thirty. Later, they produced a video that described Fulford as an osteopathic maverick.[3]

Fulford played the tape for the audience. It showed Dr. Weil, the director of the School of Integrative Medicine at the University of Arizona Medical School, narrating a comparison of treatments of otitis media inflammation by an osteopathic physician, Robert Fulford, and an allopathic pediatrician, Anita Stafford, M.D. The tape included some footage of Harold Swartz, D.O., and of Fulford's Phoenix office in the Sunrise Building. There was a discussion by Fulford of the importance of the first breath, and of the cranial and sacral osteopathic manipulative treatment method.

In the film, Dr. Fulford demonstrated a treatment of a child with inflammation of the otitis media using percussive vibration with release, followed by osteopathic manipulative treatment. This was followed by questions from Dr. Weil. In response to Weil's question about how Fulford would revise the current medical education curriculum, he recommended emphasizing function over symptoms. In addition, Fulford reminisced:

> Back in the old days—the 20s—each child at birth got a good spanking and this helped initiate free respiration—opened the respiratory mechanism.

Today that would lead to [a] suit. But with the percussion vibrator, you can spank them without being sued.

In 1929, and the Depression, I could not afford medical school, but in 1935-6, I was finally able. I was called to the Dean's office and told that I would make a better dentist than a doctor. Well, it is our aim to make clear to the medical community that they made a mistake.

About his experiences with Dr. Sutherland and their impact on his methods and outlook, Fulford commented:

We tried to absorb his teaching, but it didn't take well. I left The Cranial Academy, went to Philadelphia, studied with Dr. Arbuckle, and got a degree of understanding of stress bands of the dura mater and really understood the cranial concept. So I was not a faithful member, but after two or three years, I rejoined The Cranial Academy and have been a fairly reliable member since then. I accept Dr. Sutherland's statement that we are a spiritual and a mental being, expressing ourselves in the physical body, and until we understand the depth of that, we will not do much cranial work.

When I start to manipulate the health of the spiritual body, then the physical body changes for me.

Two years ago a professor from the colleges called me saying, "Will you please see me?" Begging for help, [he said that] he had been treated by this one and that one in the hospital. His body had been shut down, no motion. I said, "Get ready, I will treat you with twenty-first century medicine." I used my crystal into his lung area and with it pulled out the shock of the auto accident seventeen years before. He felt energy flow.

Dr. Fulford described the amount of work involved in treating patients. He said that he had to explore various kinds of vibrators, the first being oscillating types, which did not work. He related that the postman brought a brochure describing the Foredom Percussion Vibrator, and when he saw the picture, his inner self knew that was what he had been looking for. From then on, he gradually developed his technique. "I got letters from other doctors, including one that said 'quack, quack, quack.' Many physicians did not like what I was doing . . . so I tried harder."

Fulford described cases, including one of a 46-year-old nurse who hurt her back:

I came to the conclusion she was disappointed and had closed up the door to her heart. We opened it, turned her on the table and the shift in her pelvis was automatic. What mattered was the letter I got from her asking what I had done to let her body release itself. I asked what had happened to close herself up in her soul.

This is work based on research. The things we mention regarding percussion have been researched at Princeton, Yale, UCLA, Ohio State University—they are not off my head.

The book [*Dr. Fulford's Touch of Life* [4]] was published in Japan, and the editor knew a woman who had dental work in her mouth [and] was not able to open [it]. She asked for my help. We decided she needed a good spanking—we used the percussion to release it. I could tell stories by the hour.

From my friend in Maryland with an engineering degree, we report some of the cranial theories. I have followed Dr. Burr's work (1939 at Yale) regarding the knowledge we should know about voltages and patterns in the body. He noted each age had its own electrical or "L" field.

Fulford then proceeded to show a tape of Marcel Vogel, who cited Baxter's work with plants. He then described the use of crystals, coupled with the practitioner's thoughts about "pulsed breath," for coherently passing the vibration.

Continuing with this theme, Fulford described the "tree of life" as the inspiration for shaping the crystal. He described the similarity of the bonding angles of water to those of quartz, and the capacity of water to retain the information found in thoughts. He said he could measure suggestions made in the presence of water by means of absorption spectroscopy, that is, the thought transformed the water.

Fulford's final comments were a plea to participate in the understanding of patients from the "energy point of view." He felt that if this were not done, the work would fall to others outside the osteopathic profession.

• • •

There is much conceptual elision in this talk. Having retrospectively read his sources, I believe that I understand the chain of his ideas presented here.

165

Biologic matter is composed to a significant extent of water. Water has physical and energetic properties. The energetic properties can be influenced by thoughts, good and bad. Besides the similarity (I am told) in the bond angles (microscopic structure) of water molecules and quartz crystals, Vogel's refined crystals—especially those with six or seven sides—had a bond angle similar to the water molecule, and could act as a catalyst to enhance the energetic effects of thoughts or intentions in the healing process.

Metaphysically, the Tree of Life, mentioned in Judeo-Christian scripture, is further described in the later Kabbalah, Jewish wisdom writings, which has many levels of meaning. In modern times, Caroline Myss and Marcel Vogel, among others, have noted the similarity in the diagrammatic form of the Tree of Life from the Kabbalah with that of the quartz crystal.

Fulford could accept this rationale in light of Walter Russell's cosmology of the coextension of thought, light, and matter.

REFERENCES

1. During the talk, Fulford singled out his appreciation for the help given to him by Richard Koss. Fulford said that without his kindness, he would not be present at the conference.

2. While he was adamant about the nonexistence of the CRI, he never clarified, to my knowledge, exactly what he thought people were palpating. My interpretation is that it was an epiphenomenon of the flow of energy in the life field upon which observable respiration also depends.

3. Weil A. *Robert Fulford: An Osteopathic Alternative* (video). Tucson: University of Arizona, 1986.

4. Fulford RC. *Dr. Fulford's Touch of Life*. New York: Pocket Books, 1996.

APPENDIX C

# Fulford's Final Presentation
# to the Profession: Day Two

Dr. Fulford used his presentation during the second day of The Cranial Academy Convention to demonstrate his latest methods. Richard Koss, D.O., assisted Dr. Fulford to the podium, and Margaret Sorrel, D.O., volunteered to be the patient. The following is a reasonable account of the text of Dr. Fulford's speech, based on my own notes. He began:

> I want to share with you a technique—the latest research that you will not have seen anywhere else. The patient has been treated before for a pelvic problem without complete results.

Standing behind, with the patient on the table, he noted that the pelvis was up on the left, revealing a problem with the east-west axis of the body. He tested the shoulder motion and noted "something different in the shoulders." When he abducted and raised the arm, he noted a limitation at about 135° from neutral, and repeated his famous aphorism: "Problem getting into the cookie jar." In addition, he noted a head restriction to the left.

167

With the patient lying on her back, Fulford palpated the anterior-superior iliac spine bilaterally. He noted little movement in the pelvis, restriction of the abdominal diaphragm, restriction of the ribs in the upper chest, inability to take a full breath, and movement in the zygomas, but not in the parietals. He covered the patient to keep her warm from the air-conditioning, and then remarked:

> This is the latest research from Norm Shealy and Caroline Myss, the former a neurosurgeon, the latter an intuitive healer, as published in *Subtle Energies* the previous year.[1] It is elsewhere referred to as "opening the heart door."

He took a crystal, squeezed it, and charged it by rubbing with his thumb until it made a noise. He then pronounced, "The crystal is alive." He put his thoughts into the crystal and began a circular motion, similar to the method used by Marcel Vogel, saying "This is called the 'Ring of Fire,' referring to the ring of volcanic activity of the earth, corresponding to us in the endocrine organ." He started moving in a circular motion, lateral to the trunk and crossing at the pubic bones and the crown in a counter-clockwise direction, five times, then in a clockwise direction five times. He cleared the crystal with four breaths (also a technique of Vogel's), once for each facet of the crystal, and then rechecked the patient's pelvic motion: "Okay, the diaphragm is okay. You can get into the cookie jar. Lie down. You have freedom, but we will stretch [you] a little bit."

With the patient seated, Fulford did gentle myofascial release, rotating the neck. "Now we will balance the hemispheres." Standing before the seated patient, Fulford's hands were placed over the temporal squama, with the patient's hands on his arms until his hands were "thrown off." He wiggled his fingers nimbly although he was very aged.

Fulford instructed the patient to "talk to them [the audience] if you want to." Margaret responded that during the counterclockwise and clockwise rotations of the crystal, she felt a tightening of the fascia of the trunk on the respective sides that ended "in balance" back to the midline: "I heard a noise as the crystal passed my ear, a woody-woody sound, woosh-woosh." She felt motion in her pelvis, plus two distinct respiratory releases, and with each release, she felt more vitality and energy.

"Thank you very much."

At this point, Dr. Fulford said:

> This comment may not be in order, but it is what I feel. The future of med-
> icine is energy medicine, and unless The Cranial Academy does research in
> this area, the medical profession will take it over.

There followed a discussion with Dr. Koss and a reference to the video-
tape by Andrew Weil presented the day before, as well as to Ron Carson
and the availability of Vogel Crystals. It was also noted that Fulford and
Ed Slattery, D.O., had spent some time with Vogel.

> Life energy has been used by civilization for four thousand years. We need
> to develop instruments to measure this, and also need to build yourself up
> with plenty of life energy in order to be able to give it. When given energy,
> the body relaxes and feels better, which is what your patients want. How do
> you charge yourself with life energy?

He went on to discuss the intention to heal—the healing power of
osteopathy—and love. Fulford claimed validity for his ideas through his
association with Marcel Vogel, a unique and capable individual and a former research scientist for IBM.

When he was questioned about how he energized himself, Fulford
answered, "Letting the life energy run through your body, arising early,
and using the exercises in the book."[2] Regarding the door of the heart,
Fulford said he had been circulating this energy for forty years and recently hit the imprint of an old accident, which made his chemistry go hay-
wire.

He was asked who else should they read, and he answered, "Whatever
is compatible with you, including, for example, Harold Burr's *Blueprint for
Immortality*[3] on the electric pattern of life. Burr was a neuroanatomist
from Yale 1938-72." He also discussed Pranayama and how it differed
from regenerative breath. Finally, when asked how the study of osteopathy related to the use of the crystal, he replied, "How can you be successful without the knowledge of osteopathy for diagnosis and the appreciation of structure and function?"

# APPENDIX C

## REFERENCES

1. Schealy N, Myss C. The ring of fire and dhea: a theory for energetic restoration of adrenal reserves. *Subtle Energies and Energy Medicine* 1996;6(2):167-75.

2. See Appendix E.

3. Burr HS. *Blueprint for Immortality.* Essex, England: Neville Spearman, 1972.

# APPENDIX D

# Selections from Dr. Fulford's Case Files

The following are additional selections from Dr. Fulford's case files. As previously noted, each record was kept on one eight by nine-and-a-half inch sheet with cursory notes written by hand. They were selected from the last seven years of Dr. Fulford's life to reflect the mature synthesis of his work, and to demonstrate the variety of complaints that he treated, and the diagnoses and treatment approaches that he utilized. At times the notes are terse—Doc was getting old. He kept a keen focus in treatment but was less concerned about communicating through his notes. Also, as he himself admitted, his reserve of energy to treat was limited, and he therefore relied heavily on the use of the percussion vibrator.

Italics reflect the author's editorial comments; otherwise, the material is presented just as it appeared in the case record.

## CASE 1: J.H. 24-year-old male; no complaint specified

HISTORY

Patient fell through the floor and caught himself on rafters with arms spread out. Age 10.

At fourteen and eight while swimming he hit his head. Eight months ago had jaw surgery.

Pain in neck seems to space out. Hard to study. On homeopathic medicine. Deep sleeper.

Difficult first three months of life. Mouth breather. Fell off horse age three. Chicken pox.

EXAMINATION

No skull motion, depression right side of skull.

Neck tense. Rigid rib cage, shallow breather.

No motion in pelvis, right hip—no rotation in right leg.

Arm raise restricted on left 110 degrees.

DIAGNOSIS

Incomplete breath at birth. Accidents increased breathing difficulty. Depressed thymus gland.

TREATMENT

Percussed right trochanter—released thymus. Percussed left shoulder—released pelvis.

Percussed spine and right partietal.

Patient able to deep breathe; do exercises.

EDITOR'S COMMENTS

*Patient seen one time, was charged $25, but paid $100.*

*Fulford also worked out the patient's signs based on the time and date of birth—something he did regularly.*

## CASE 2: A.S. 2-month-old female; problems with nursing

HISTORY

Pregnancy had spotting at 21 weeks. Delivery: 2/14 labor—2/15 epidural 20 min. (labor difficulty implied).

Right clavicle fracture. Drugs.

Cries for unknown reason, nursing problem, jaundice.

EXAMINATION

Narrow right nostril, right arm raise restricted. Rib cage rigid. Breathing to diaphragm. Right leg restricted in rotation; torsion of right knee. Right fibula restricted.

DIAGNOSIS

Incomplete breath. Right vagus restricted in neck.

TREATMENT

Magnet north pole to umbilicus and sacrum. Release the right arm and leg. Breath. Percussed right knee and ankle. Magnet south pole to parietals. Complete change in baby.

EDITOR'S COMMENTS

*Was seen once in follow up at six months due to recurrent otitis media and was re-treated without details specified.*

## CASE 3: A.C. 3-year-old female; parents complain she walks on her toes

HISTORY

Child walks on toes, not talking, falls to stop, forward position in motion.

Pregnancy, no problems.

Delivery normal labor, no complications. Nursed 12 weeks; crawled at 9 months, walked at 14 months.

Accidents: fell down steps when 2 years old.

EXAMINATION

Very hard to examine. Wouldn't lie on table. Skull very tight frontal ridge. Tension in left rib cage. No motion in pelvis. Left leg had no motion in the hip socket.

Attached report MRI of the head from Johns Hopkins University Hospital indicated defuse delayed myelinization of frontal and occipital white matter, also in the posterior limb of the posterior capsule. Atrophy of the corpus collosum was noted. EEG showed pattern consistent with seizure disorder of multi-focal origin.

### DIAGNOSIS

Incomplete first breath at birth, partial spastic.

### TREATMENT

Percussed left knee, right trochanter, sacrum, spine. Reestablished motion in left leg and hip. Motion returned to the skull; child was able to walk on feet when finished.

### EDITOR'S COMMENTS

*Patient was seen 15 times over three years. Treatment included percussion, cranial osteopathic manipulation, and, on one occasion, magnets applied to the umbilicus. After the third treatment the body seemed to begin progressive relaxation of spasticity.*

## CASE 4: J.N. 14-year-old male complaining of back problems

### HISTORY

Complaining of back problems. Has reading problems—eyes (?)

Knees—Osgood Schlatters.

Pregnancy normal.

Delivery forceps, oxygen. Nursed for 10 months, born with left leg turned in, casted. Had chicken pox, sinus.

Accident: over the handle bars age 7, injury to teeth.

Plays soccer.

### EXAMINATION

No motion in skull. Frozen pelvis. e.g. won't turn in hip sockets. Torsion in left knee. No motion in lower spine.

DIAGNOSIS

Frozen pelvis due to casting of left leg at birth.

TREATMENT

Release the skull, which freed motion in the hip sockets. Percussed left knee, trochanters, sacrum, spine, umbilicus.

EDITOR'S COMMENTS

*Patient seen 10 times over two years, had fracture to arch of the foot, compensated with an arch support. Fulford's notes include "severe pain in hamstrings; lower leg in a twist; body responded to percussion."*

## CASE 5: J. A. 6-year-old male, hyperactive

HISTORY

Child very active, on Mellaril.

Pregnancy, morning sickness most of nine months.

Delivery : six hours, no problems.

Accidents: Had a bad fall at seven or eight months.

EXAMINATION

Tight skull, arm raises right and left to 100 degrees. Sternal angle fixed. Tight ribs (diaphragm), frozen pelvis, torsion left knee. Restriction of hip sockets. Shallow breaths.

DIAGNOSIS

Incomplete breath at birth and due to fall (see letter).

TREATMENT

Percussed left knee, sacrum, spine, sternal angle, occipital protuberance, cranial treatment.

EDITOR'S COMMENTS

*Attached was a draft of a letter, written on an AAO Convocation program page, in response to the referring physician's letter:*

Dear Dr. M.,

I wish to thank you for allowing me to share in the treatment of J.A.

*Examination*

No membranous motion in the skull; arm raise 100 degrees in left and right arm. No motion in the rib cage at the level of the diaphragm. Pelvis was frozen. Very little motion in the hip sockets. Torsion in left knee. These findings gave the following explanation to the child's problem.

The lack of membranous motion indicates that the synchronization of the lungs and heart didn't take place at the time of the first breath, which would establish the rhythm in the brain.

The arm raise is telling that the scapulae are stuck to the ribs so a fixation at the sternal angle, 4th dorsal vertebrae. With the upper four ribs were in a fixed position. The tightness at the level of the diaphragm is shown by history of lack of bowel movement for 5 days. This is telling the Solar Plexus of nerves are in distress.

The frozen pelvis is telling that the respiratory wave of the first breath didn't penetrate down to the sacrum. The tight hips are part of the pelvic problem.

*Treatment*

First was percussion on the right rib cage to release the diaphragm. (Here is where relationship is important. The knee, diaphragm and neck are a unit. Similar to the proton-neutron-electron of the atom.) The diaphragm is the neuter field and magnet. The knee and the neck are electric so if the neuter field (diaphragm) is dormant the knee and neck can't function. With diaphragm and the solar plexus inhibited, the end result is pelvic stagnation or "frozen." The torsion in knee is a diaphragm problem.

After percussion on the rib cage, I went to the inner surface of the left knee and good release. The mother helped to hold child down, heard the noise of the bones snap as they shifted in the pelvis.

The next percussion was the sacro-coxygeal angle with my hand over the umbilicus. (Reason palpating hand on the umbilicus, the primitive groove and primitive streak form part of the perineum and goes up to the umbilicus.) Percussed over the 5th lumbar and other hand on the umbilicus. Felt the wave come into pelvis.

Percussed spine. When I got to the 4th thoracic it was tight and finally loose as though it was dry bones. Percussed the 7th cervical, hand on the head, the occipital protuberance. (I hold head down and steady.)

Check child breathing going through the rib cage and abdomen and some rhythm in the occipital area.

*That ended first day. Second day:*

Mother reported good sleep, breathing easy and stomach moving with breathing.

Percussed inner surface of right knee (treat effect midline axis) the sacrum, spine (there is a problem in the spine at or around the lumbo dorsal junction), sternal angle.

Percussed deltoid recess of the left arm and palpating hand on the sphenoid or forehead—got motion. Hand on skull got a flip of membranes of which the mother heard the snap. That ended treatment.

Then answered questions of the mother. Then prescribed magnet. Get magnet at Radio Shack. Snap negative pole to the sole of the feet every night for 2 hours. (The magnet will stimulate the L field and help bring the physical body around.)

The child's right foot is turned outward. Don't be concerned. That is caused by a disturbance of the sub occipital muscle. Once the neck livens up, I told mother that it takes one month for every year its been in. So in six months some changes would show up.

My suggestion of treatment every two weeks for two months, then every month. Percuss the area suggested on second day.

## CASE 6: N.L. 10-year-old male with a behavior problem

HISTORY

Child is on Ritalin, behavior problems, socially, etc. Attention spasm. Disposition poor.

Pregnancy: stressful—anxiety—conflict (financial).

Baby tossed up by father.

DELIVERY

Unable to vaginally—so C-section done. Labor was induced.

Infection: tonsillitis—chicken pox.

Accident: dived off pool and head hit mother's face, age 3. In a store, pulled bath rack over on him, age 4. Broke right leg.

8 years old, broke left forearm.

EXAMINATION

No motion right leg—torsion right knee, locked ankle. Torsion pattern in pelvis—mid dorsal spine curves. Right arm raise 170 degrees, left normal. Left forearm rotary motion limited. Head rotation to right limited. No motion in skull; frontal overlap.

DIAGNOSIS

Right leg motion restricted due to broke tibia, left arm lack of motion due to broken forearm. Rigid skull due to accident at 3 years of age.

TREATMENT

Percussed right knee, tibia and fibula in the ankle. Percussed left forearm, spine, and sternum. Crystal to forehead to release skull, then manipulated skull.

EDITOR'S COMMENTS

*Patient seen one time.*

## CASE 7: E.A. 5-month-old female with congenital hip displacement

HISTORY

Left hip displaced, no success with traction.

Pregnancy: morning sickness.

Delivery: quick, good cry, nursed about 5 hours later.

Baby rolls over, not crawling.

EXAMINATION

No rotation in left femur; some restriction in right femur.

Tight rib cage on left. Left arm raise limited. Torsion in left knee. Restriction of ankle.

DIAGNOSIS

Misalignment of left femur, due to torsion of left knee.

TREATMENT

Percussed left knee and ankle. Sacrum, spine, left shoulder. Cranial manipulation. Home exercises—push on both feet.

EDITOR'S COMMENTS

*Patient seen three times over three months. On third visit, note under examination says "hip normal."*

## Case 8: N.B. 10-year-old female with allergies since infancy

HISTORY

Allergies since a baby.

Pregnancy: sick 4th and 5th months.

Delivery: difficult, didn't breath right away, became purple, requiring oxygen.

Sick: dermatitis, eczema.

Accidents: none.

EXAMINATION

No motion in the skull, head-turn to the left limited.
Arm raise right 120 degrees, left 110 degrees.
Rigid rib cage, no pelvic motion. Torsion of left knee.

DIAGNOSIS

Incomplete breath at birth.

TREATMENT

Percussed left knee, sacrum, spine, rib cage, base of skull, sternal angle.
Breathing exercises.

EDITOR'S COMMENTS

*Patient seen once.*

## CASE 9: K.B. 12-year-old female with constant sore throat

HISTORY

Constant sore throat.
Pregnancy: no problems.
Delivery easy, nursed.
Sick: ear infections.
Accidents: 16 months of age fell down steps, stitches in chin.

EXAMINATION

Very tight skull. Rib cage tight, torsion in pelvis. Mouth breather.

DIAGNOSIS

Incomplete breath due to the fall.

TREATMENT

Percussed sacrum, spine, right parietal, sternal angle. Got release in the
skull.
Breathing exercises.

EDITOR'S COMMENTS

*Patient seen one time.*

# APPENDIX E

# Daily Supplemental Exercises

These exercises were developed to maintain and augment the vital force within. Done daily, these exercises will assure that the beneficial effects brought about by your treatments are maintained. Though these exercises are straightforward and simple, they have profound effect. Doing these daily and properly will help assure you of better health and increased vitality.

1. **Breathing**  Sitting up straight and comfortably, place the tongue just above the two front teeth on the ridge on the roof of the palate. Close mouth and inhale through your nostrils, fully expanding your lungs and hold for the count of seven. Exhale through the mouth, at your own rate, keeping the tongue touching the palate.

   Do this for 7 breaths twice a day.

   This is considered the most important exercise.

2. **Arm Raising from Standing**
   **a.** Stand with your feet shoulder-width apart, with arms extended out to the sides at shoulder height (Fig. 1a-c).

**b.** Left palm should face upward and the right palm should face downward.

**c.** Hold this position for as long as possible, breathing full deep breaths. The ideal length of time is 5-10 minutes.

**d.** At the end of the exercise, keeping the arms straight, slowly raise them up and out to the sides of the body and above the head, not letting the arms come forward (Fig. 1d). Then lower the arms.

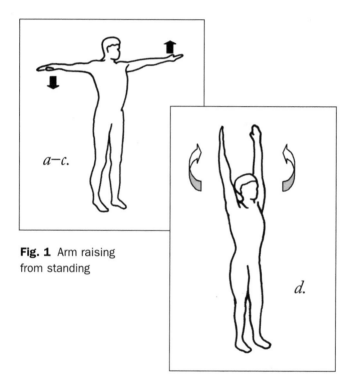

*a–c.*

*d.*

**Fig. 1** Arm raising from standing

**3. Hip Twist**   Lie on your back with your arms stretched out to your side at shoulder height with the left palm facing up and the right palm facing down.

Bring the feet together with knees straight.

Lift the left leg off the floor, keeping the left leg straight, and roll the left hip and left leg over the right leg (Fig. 2).

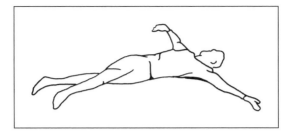

**Fig. 2** Hip twist

Keep both shoulders on the floor and breathe fully while holding the position for up to 5 minutes or until you feel pain. Do until you are able to hold for 5 minutes without pain.

Bring the left leg back to the original position and do the same procedure for the right leg.

Hold the positions for 5 minutes or until pain is felt on each side, once a day. Ideally the exercise should be done without experiencing pain.

4. **Spinal Stretch**  Sit in an upright chair so that your thighs are parallel with the floor and the lower part of the leg is perpendicular to the floor.

Bend over, place the elbows on the inside of your knees.

Turn your palms away from each other and tuck your fingers under the arch of each foot while placing your thumb over the top of the foot. Let your spine fully stretch in this position (Fig 3).

Breathe slowly and fully for up to 5 minutes. Do once a day.

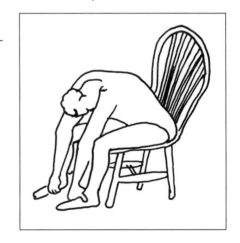

**Fig. 3** Spinal stretch

183

**5. Standing**   Stand against a wall so that your heels, lower back, and the spine between your shoulder blades and the back of your head touch the wall.

Raise the arms straight out in front of you with your thumbs touching (Fig. 4a). Then, as slowly as you can, raise them straight above your head, finally touching the wall (Fig. 4b).

Then lower the arms out and down at your sides.

Again, remember to breathe slowly and fully.

Do this two times, once a day.

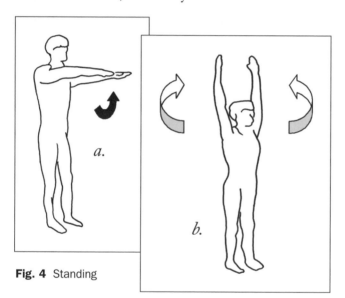

**Fig. 4** Standing

**6. Shoulder Rolls**

Sit in a chair with your back straight and both feet placed on the floor.

**a.** Bend your elbows in front of you and let your fingertips rest on the tops of your shoulders (Fig. 5a).

**b.** Breathe slowly and fully. On inhalation, lift your elbows up toward the ceiling and lower your head down (Fig. 5b).

**c.** On exhalation, roll the elbows out to the side and back to the starting position (Fig. 5a) while lifting the head back (Fig. 5c).

Do steps **a.–c.** 5 times, 2-3 times a day.

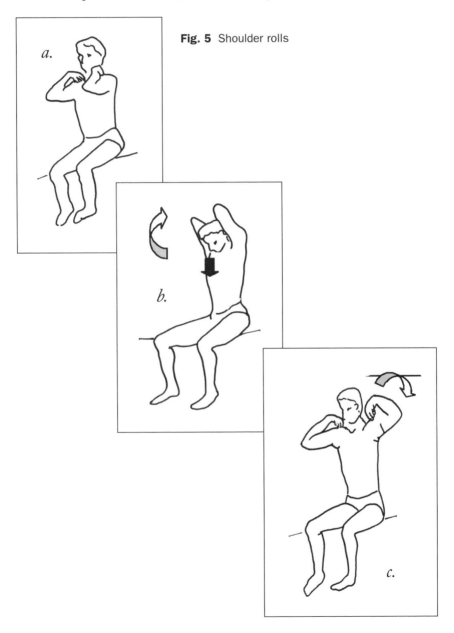

**Fig. 5** Shoulder rolls

**7. Knee Bend**   Stand four to five feet from the wall and face it, with your feet shoulder-width apart, and your palms on the wall at shoulder height.

Bend your knees as much as possible while still keeping your heels on the floor (Fig. 6).

While knees are bent, breathe fully for one minute.

Repeat 5 times, once a day.

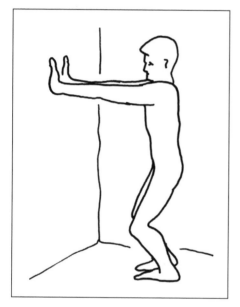

**Fig. 6** Knee bend

APPENDIX F

# Bibliography

Arbuckle BE. *The Selected Writings of Beryl E. Arbuckle.* Camp Hill, PA: National Osteopathic Institute and Cerebral Palsy Foundation, 1977.

Ayala F, Dobzhansky T (eds.) *Studies in the Philosophy of Biology.* Berkeley: University of California Press, 1974.

Bach E. *Heal Thyself: An Explanation of the Real Cause and Cure of Disease.* London: C.W. Daniel Co., Ltd., 1978 (orig. 1931).

Bailey A. *Esoteric Healing.* New York: Lucis Publishing Company, 1991.

Becker R. *The Body Electric: Electromagnetism and the Foundation of Life.* New York: William Morrow, 1987.

Bel F. William Garner Sutherland át-il été influencé par Walter Russell. *Apostil* (Academie d'Osteopathie de France) 2000;6:14-22.

Bergson H. *Creative Evolution.* New York: Henry Holt, 1911.

Burr HS. *Blueprint for Immortality.* Essex, England: Neville Spearman, 1972.

Campbell C (ed.) *The Osteopathic Technique of John Wernham* (video with diagrams). Maidstone, England: Institute of Classical Osteopathy, 1996.

Chaitow L. *Cranial Manipulation Theory and Practice.* Kent, England: Churchill-Livingston, 1999.

Chamberlain D. *Babies Remember Birth.* Los Angeles: Jeremy Tarcher, Inc., 1988.

Chila A. "Fascial-ligamentous Release." In *Foundations for Osteopathic Medicine,* Ward R. (ed.) Baltimore: Williams and Wilkins, 1997.

Clark G. *The Man Who Tapped the Secrets of the Universe.* Waynesboro, VA: Walter Russell Foundation, 1956.

Comeaux Z. Facilitated oscillatory release – a method of dynamic assessment and treatment of somatic dysfunction. *AAO Journal,* in press.

Comeaux Z. The role of vibration and oscillation in the development of osteopathic thought. *AAO Journal* 2000;10(3):19–24.

Cunningham FG et al. (eds.) *Williams Obstetrics,* 20th ed. Stamford, CT: Appleton and Lang, 1997.

Diamond J. *Life Energy.* New York: Dodd Mead, 1985.

Dillaway N. *Consent.* Lee's Summit, MO: Utility Press, 1967.

Dingle E. *Breathing Your Way to Youth.* Yucca Valley, CA: The Institute of Mental Physics, 1931.

Dorman T. *Prolotherapy in the Lumbar Spine and Pelvis.* Philadelphia: Hanley and Belfus, 1995.

Dossey L. *Healing Words.* New York: Harper Collins, 1993.

Dossey L. *Prayer is Good Medicine.* San Francisco: Harper, 1996.

Dossey L. *Reinventing Medicine: Beyond Mind-Body to the New Era of Healing.* San Francisco: Harper, 1999.

Dreisch H. *The History and Theory of Vitalism.* London: MacMillan and Co., 1914.

Eklund G, Hagbarth K. Normal variability of tonic vibration reflexes in man. *Experimental Neurology.* 1966;16:80-92.

Friedman H, Gilliar W, Glassman J. *Myofascial and Fascial-Ligamentous Approaches in Osteopathic Manipulative Medicine.* San Francisco: San Francisco International Manual Medicine Society, 2000: 6.

Fryette H. *Principles of Osteopathic Technique.* Indianapolis, IN: American Academy of Osteopathy, 1994 (orig. 1954).

Frymann V. Unpublished address notes, 2000 International Symposium on Traditional Osteopathy, Montreal, Canada.

Fulford R. *Basic and Advanced Percussion Course Notebooks.* Unpublished, but may become available from The Cranial Academy.

Fulford R. *Dr. Fulford's Touch of Life.* New York: Pocket Books, 1996.

Hebb D. *The Organization of Behavior.* New York: Wiley, 1942.

Hoffman H. *Esoteric Osteopathy.* Philadelphia: self-published, 1908.

Hunt V. *Infinite Mind: Science of the Human Vibration of Consciousness.* Malibu, CA: Malibu Publishing Co., 1989.

Jealous J. *Emergence of Originality: A Biodynamic View of Osteopathy in the Cranial Field.* Franconia, NH: self-published (no date provided).

Johnston B. *New Age Healing.* Havant Hants, England: self-published, 1975.

Johnston W. *Functional Methods.* Indianapolis, IN: American Academy of Osteopathy, 1994.

Jones L. *Jones Strain Counterstrain,* 2nd ed. Boise, ID: Jones Strain-Countertrain Inc., 1995.

Kappler R. *Foundations for Osteopathic Medicine.* Baltimore: Williams and Wilkins, 1997.

Kelso JA. *Dynamic Patterns: The Self-Organization of Brain and Behavior.* Cambridge, MA: MIT Press, 1995.

Korr I. *The Collected Papers of Irvin M. Korr.* Indianapolis, IN: American Academy of Osteopathy, 1979.

Littlejohn JM. *The Fundamentals of Osteopathic Technique.* Maidstone, England: Institute of Classical Osteopathy, 1975.

Leboyer F. *Birth Without Violence.* New York: Alfred Knopf, 1975.

Magoun H. *Osteopathy in the Cranial Field,* 3d ed. Indianapolis, IN: The Cranial Academy, 1976.

Maigne R. *Diagnosis and Treatment of Pain of Vertebral Origin.* Baltimore: Williams and Wilkins, 1996.

Miguel A. Hebb's dream: the resurgence of cell assemblies. *Neuron* 1997;19:219–21.

Mitchell F. *The Muscle Energy Manual,* vol. 1. East Lansing, MI: MET Press, 1995.

Montalenti G. "From Aristotle to Democritus via Darwin." In *Studies in the Philosophy of Biology,* Ayala F, Dobzhansky T (eds.) Berkeley: University of California Press, 1974.

Moskalenko Y. "Principles of Instrumental Measurement of the Efficacy of Osteopathy in the Cranial Field." Speech given at 1999 Symposium of the Deutsche Osteopathie Kolleg.

Nuccitelli R. "Endogenous Electric Fields in Developing Embryos." In *Electromagnetic Fields,* Blank M. (ed.) Washington, D.C.: American Chemical Society, 1995: 109.

O'Connell, J. *Bioelectric Fascial Activation and Release.* Indianapolis, IN: American Academy of Osteopathy, 2000.

Patterson M. A model mechanism for spinal segmental facilitation. *JAOA* 1976;76:62-72.

Pert C. *Molecules of Emotion: Why You Feel the Way You Feel.* New York: Scribner, 1997.

Reich W. *Selected Writings: An Introduction to Orgonomy.* New York: Farrar, Straus, Giroux, 1973.

Richards D, McMillin D, Mein E, Nelspon C. Osteopathic regulation of physiology. *AAO Journal* 2000;11(3):34-8.

Roll JP, Gilhodes JC. Proprioceptive sensory codes mediating movement trajectory perception: human hand vibration-induced drawing illusions. *Canadian Journal of Physiology Pharmacology* 1995;73:295-304.

Russell W. *The Message of the Divine Iliad,* vol. 1. Waynesboro, VA: University of Science and Philosophy, 1948.

Russell W. *The Universal One.* Waynesboro, VA: University of Science and Philosophy, 1974 (orig. 1926).

Sakumarai Y. Population coding of cell assemblies—what is in the brain? *Neuroscience Research* 1996;26(1):1–16.

Samsonvich A, McNaughton B. Path propagation and cognitive mapping in a continuous attractor neural network model. *Journal of Neuroscience* 1997;17(15):5900–20.

Schalow G, Zach G. Neuronal reorganization through oscillator formation training in patients with cns lesions. *Journal of the Peripheral Nervous System,* 1998;3:165-88.

Schealy N, Myss C. The ring of fire and dhea: a theory for energetic restoration of adrenal reserves. *Subtle Energies and Energy Medicine* 1996;6(2):167.

Sergueef N, Nekson K, Glonek T. Changes in the traube-herring wave following cranial manipulation. *AAO Journal* 2001;11(1):17-19.

Spatz H. Hebb's concept of synaptic plasticity and neuronal cell assemblies. *Behavior Brain Research* 1996:78(1):3–7.

Spencer H. *First Principles.* New York: A. L. Burt Publishing, 1880.

Still AT. *Philosophy and Mechanical Principles of Osteopathy.* Kansas City: Hudson-Kimberly Publishing Co., 1902.

Still AT. *Autobiography of A.T. Still.* Indianapolis, IN: American Academy of Osteopathy, 1981 (orig. 1897, 1908).

Still AT. *Philosophy of Osteopathy.* Indianapolis, IN: American Association of Osteopathy, 1977 (orig. 1899).

Still AT. *Osteopathy: Research and Practice.* Seattle: Eastland Press, 1992 (orig. 1910).

Stone R. *Polarity Therapy,* vols. 1 and 2. Sebastopol, CA: CRCS Publications, 1987 (orig. 1954).

Sutherland WG. *Contributions of Thought.* Fort Worth, TX: Sutherland Cranial Teaching Foundation, 1967.

Sutherland WG. *The Cranial Bowl.* Indianapolis, IN: The Cranial Academy, 1948 (orig. 1939).

Sutherland WG. *Teachings in the Science of Osteopathy.* Fort Worth, TX: Sutherland Cranial Teaching Foundation, 1990 (reprinted from the 1949 Yearbook of the Academy of Applied Osteopathy).

**191**

Trowbridge C. *Andrew Taylor Still 1828–1917*. Kirksville, MO: Thomas Jefferson University Press, 1991.

Tompkins T. *The Secret Life of Plants*. New York: Avon, 1974.

Truby W. The newborn baby's cry. *Acta Paediatrica Scandinavica* 1965 (supp.): 163.

Typaldos S. *Orthopathic Medicine: The Unification of Orthopedics and Osteopathy through the Fascial Distortion Model*. Brewer, ME: Orthopathic Global Press, 1997.

Upledger JE, Vredevoogd J. *Craniosacral Therapy*. Chicago: Eastland Press, 1983.

Varela FJ. Resonant cell assemblies: a new approach to cognitive functions and neuronal synchrony. *Biological Research* 1995;28(1):81-95.

Van Buskirk R. *The Still Technique Manual*. Indianapolis, IN: American Academy of Osteopathy, 1999.

Van Buskirk R. Nociceptive reflex and somatic dysfunction, a model. *JAOA*, 1990;90(9):792.

Verny T. *The Secret Life of the Unborn Child*. New York: Dell Publishing, 1981.

Vogel M. Miscellaneous tapes and newsletters from Psychic Research, Inc., San Jose, CA (now closed). Check availability through Lifestream Associates, 70 Sable Court, Winter Springs, FL 32708.

Von Reichenbach K. *The Odic Force*, O'Byrne F (trans.) San Diego: The Book Tree, 2000.

Von Reichenbach K. *Physico-Physiological Researches in the Dynamics of Magnetism, Electricity, Heat, Light, Crystallization, and Chemism as They Relate to Vital Force*. New York: J Redfield, Clinton-Hall, 1851.

Ward R. *Foundations of Osteopathic Medicine*. Baltimore: Williams and Wilkins, 1997.

Weaver C. The primary brain vesicles and the three cranial vertebra. *JAOA*, 1938;37(8): 348.

Weil A. *Robert Fulford: An Osteopathic Alternative* (video). Tucson: University of Arizona, 1986.

Weil A. *Spontaneous Healing*. New York: Alfred Knopf, 1995.

Wernham J. *The Osteopathic Techniques of John Wernham* (video), Campbell C (ed.) Maidstone, England: Institute of Classical Osteopathy, 1996.

Whitehead AN. *Science and the Modern World*. New York: New American Library, 1925.

Wilson EO. *Consilience, The Unity of Knowledge*. New York: Knopf, 1998.

Zink JG. Respiratory and circulatory care, the conceptual model. *Osteopathic Annals* 1977;5(3):108-12.

# Index